contents

Chapter 1: **Why blood-sugar control is vital**
In this chapter we look at some fundamental stuff about how your body uses different kinds of foods, and why blood sugar balance is key to weight and health.

Chapter 2: **Body Composition**
Now we move on to understanding that what your body looks like on the outside doesn't necessarily match how it functions on the inside.

Chapter 3: **Nutrition**
We are really getting down to the nitty gritty. Let's take a closer look at nutrients: what are they, why you need them, and where to get them!

Chapter 4: **Creating your unique food plan**
Everything to help you create your own unique eating plan is here!

Chapter 5: **Other lifestyle factors**
It isn't just food that affects your weight and health. In this section we will explore the role of exercise and stress.

Chapter 6: **Living in the real world**
This chapter explores some emotional issues about food and social eating.

the 6 diet
food combat for **diabetes**

Elaine Wilson

Fisher King Publishing

the 6 diet

ISBN 978-1-906377-72-4
Copyright © Elaine Wilson 2014

Published by
Fisher King Publishing
The Studio
Arthington Lane
Pool-in-Wharfedale
LS21 1JZ
England

Remembering Ivy Moore.
She died too soon.

Preface

Diabetes? The philosophy behind my approach to diabetes is 'less means more means better'. This simple wisdom is the foundation of RebalanceDiabetes: less medication, less body fat, less fear, less chance of developing complications normally associated with diabetes such as pain, heart disease, amputations, blindness leading to more control, more confidence, more energy, leading to better blood sugar balance, better body image, better health, better quality of life. Lots of people have already experienced the many benefits of the RebalanceDiabetes dietary and lifestyle programme. They got great results. You can too.

The best way to control your blood sugar is through food – eating the right foods in the right quantities to meet your own individual body and lifestyle needs.

The best way to control your weight is through food – ensuring that what you eat protects and enhances your own unique body composition: making certain the weight you lose is fat.

The best way to prevent or manage your diabetes is through food. Simply that. And it isn't rocket science. A few simple guidelines will reap immediate benefits. A well-devised personalised dietary plan will reap immense benefits. It will help you to successfully control your blood sugar, lose abdominal fat that is so clearly linked now with serious illnesses including diabetes, and feel healthier and more energetic.

This book has been written with you in mind. Largely it has been written from the perspective of combating type 2 diabetes, but nonetheless blood sugar balance is a key factor for optimum health and weight loss whether you already have glycaemic health problems or not. So here I share all the information to help you, whether you have already developed and been diagnosed with diabetes – either Type 1 or 2; whether you have been diagnosed as being insulin resistant, or otherwise at risk of developing type 2 diabetes; whether you recognise that you are carrying too much dangerous abdominal fat, linked with serious illness; or whether you simply want to lose some weight in the most healthy and beneficial manner – making sure you shed fat rather than healthy lean tissue. In fact this book contains more than you possibly need to know to optimise your own health and body image!

Here's the thing: I once asked a doctor why the information given to newly diagnosed diabetics is so scant. He replied that people aren't ready for too much advice! Can it really be possible to give too much advice in the matter – without the advice how can people be able to follow it? How can they get the very best outcomes from dietary change if they are not given the very best, most complete advice?

So this book contains ALL the advice I could possibly share with you about how to balance your blood sugars, disperse abdominal fat and achieve your own optimum health and body image. It might contain more than you personally feel the need to know. That's OK – take the bits you need right now and work with them, the rest will be waiting for when you feel ready to go that step further. I make no apologies for giving you all that I have to give: you've bought my book, and you deserve an unabridged account of how to achieve the very best for yourself!

It really is easy to get great results. RebalanceDiabetes is an education programme devised to combat diabetes. It was established in 2013 to provide quality diet and lifestyle information to help diabetic patients balance and maintain optimum blood-sugar levels; achieve and maintain healthy weight; and generally manage their condition to avoid many of the secondary problems associated with type 2 diabetes, i.e. diabetic neuropathy, cardiovascular disease, stroke etc. The programme has so far achieved great results – not just for those with type 2 diabetes, but also for some diagnosed with type 1 diabetes, and for some who just want to lose weight in the healthiest way possible.

'the 6 diet' contains all the information delivered on the RebalanceDiabetes education programme, which has helped many people to realise the benefits that you deserve for yourself.

Why 'the 6 diet' is important

Type 2 Diabetes is one of the biggest health challenges we face in the 21st century. As the mainstream press and media remind us on an almost daily basis, it is reaching epidemic proportions.

If the figures relating to the current prevalence are alarming, then the forecast for the escalation of type 2 diabetes over the next 2 decades is nothing short of terrifying:

- Estimated global prevalence for 2010 (latest figures available) is 285 million and is expected to affect 438 million people by 2030
- The International Diabetes Federation (IDF) estimated that in 2010 the five countries with the largest numbers of people with diabetes were India (over 70 million people currently diagnosed with type 2 diabetes), China, the United States (about 29 million currently diagnosed), Russia and Brazil.

- In 2013 it was reported that China tops the world scale – with 114 million people diagnosed with type 2 diabetes and 50% of the adult population showing signs of pre-diabetic insulin resistance.
- According to the charity DiabetesUK:
- In 2009 there were 2.6 million people who have been diagnosed with diabetes in the UK.
- By 2025, there will be more than four million people with diabetes in the UK.
- This is equivalent to:
    - around 400 people every day
    - almost 17 people every hour
    - three people every ten minutes
    - over 4% of the population in the UK, and rising!
- It is estimated that there are up to half a million more people in the UK who have diabetes but have not yet been diagnosed

Worryingly, health targets in the UK are not being met. Despite type 2 diabetes regularly featuring in the news, levels continue to rise.

Despite the National Institute for Clinical Excellence (NICE) issuing guidelines in 2005, recommending that all patients newly diagnosed with type 2 diabetes be offered the opportunity to take part in a structured education programme to help them manage their condition, service provision remains patchy.

'the 6 diet' is a comprehensive guide to nutrition and weight-loss *whether or not you need to combat diabetes*. It is specifically designed to help you meet the magic blood-glucose target of '6', hence its name!

In this book you will find everything you need to know about how your body processes different nutrient types; why you need to include a wide-range of nutrients in your diet; and how to build your personalised eating plan, specifically tailored for your individual needs and lifestyle.

Praise for 'the 6 diet'

Internationally renowned nutritional writer and founder of The Institute for Optimum Nutrition, Patrick Holford, endorses **'the 6 diet'**. This is what he said:

> "**'the 6 diet'** makes good nutritional sense, applying the latest principles of optimum nutrition and low GL diet, rather than the outdated low fat, low calorie approach, coupled with the wisdom of traditional Chinese principles about vital energy, which, I believe, is a core element ignored in western approaches."

Success stories

The following are just some of the great testimonials from people who have found RebalanceDiabetes and **'the 6 diet'** beneficial to improve weight, body-shape, health and vitality:

> **Jon** says: "*I was diagnosed with type 2 diabetes several years ago, and despite my very best attempts to get my blood-sugar under control I couldn't get my levels below 16, 17, 18 or even 19 and 20 – dangerously high! I joined a gym, I followed every bit of advice from the NHS Dietician, but to no avail. My Diabetes Specialist was adamant that I MUST increase my dietary efforts. Now, thanks to Elaine's advice, just 6 weeks later my blood sugar levels typically range between 5.8 and 7 – hitting my target perfectly; I have lost 5kgs in weight; and my partner and family have all noticed that 'I am a different man!'*"

> **Simon**, diagnosed with type 1 diabetes went very public in his praise for RebalanceDiabetes:
> "*Ever since being diagnosed as diabetic, I have struggled to keep the weight off especially around my waist. There has been a tendency when experiencing low blood sugar to over compensate by overeating. With Elaine's system not only do I feel much better but the real bonus for me is that my blood sugars are so well balanced that some days I don't have to take any fast acting insulin at all!*"
> You can hear it in Simon's own words in his video testimonial on YouTube by following the link here: **https://www.youtube.com/watch?v=nknBWTZ60uQ**

"*I am feeling on top of the world. Very energetic and extremely comfortable...What do I do with my now-too-big clothes? I love it! Many thanks for your help and advice.*" - **Margaret**

"*I have gone from a ball shape to having an hour-glass figure. As of yesterday I have lost 2 stones and am absolutely delighted!*" - **Natalya**

"*I couldn't believe how quickly my body changed and also how much I was eating every day! I was never hungry and this has changed the way I think about food. It's so easy to do - I won't ever go back to the old ways – everyone should know this because it affects long term health.*" – **Andy**

"*The advice is so different from anything else out there and yet makes perfect sense. I'm over the moon with how I now feel after embracing a new way of eating and seeing the results really quickly.*" - **Nicky**

"*Elaine's unique approach to properly educating participants about food was a really enlightening journey, revealing some really big surprises and explained why despite great effort over many years and many different diets, I never lost the weight I wanted to. It makes perfect sense and introduces new thinking about how we should care for our bodies.*" - **Sarah**

"*I learned so much that I didn't know – it's the opposite of what you think you should be doing. I want to be a good weight but I also care about my health.*" – **Oksana**

"*Although I am delighted with the weight loss, what is good is that I have lost it from all the places I wanted to. Amazing, but that is not the real benefit! What the eating plan has done for me is much more. Within 2 weeks I had lost the urge to have a nap every time I sat down, and instead I have gained more energy and zest than I have had in a long time.*" - **Jane**

"I have now taken a whole lifestyle change and the course has set me on the road for a healthy diet for the rest of my life. Gone are the cravings for sweet foods, my energy levels are improving day on day and I feel and look so much better." - **Darren**

Mike, diagnosed with type 2 diabetes, says:

"Dear Elaine - Thank-you for all the advice and help you have given me while attending your RebalanceDiabetes programme. I was greatly impressed with your in depth knowledge of the treatment of diabetes from a dietary point of view.

"Having been involved with clinical advice for the past 3 years I was not moving forward in lowering my blood glucose range to an acceptable level. I was also putting weight on. Although I had been given targets of 4 to 8 I was often as high as 20 or more. Since following your advice on suitable foods and drink I am now within my target ranges and have lost two stone in weight. The NHS clinic has been very pleased with my condition. With many thanks for your help..."

Hayley has Type 1 Diabetes: *"Within just 2 weeks of starting the RebalanceDiabetes programme, my blood sugars were so well controlled that I reduced my Novorapid insulin, and have now gone from 5+ shots per. day to just 1. I always had this feeling of 'what can I eat?' This is now clear. Thank You!"*

About the Author

Elaine Wilson is a therapist with many year's experience of changing lives through the beneficial application of food and dietary principles. Patient experience and overwhelmingly positive feedback have led to the creation of **'the 6 diet'**, to bring the learning, the benefits and the positive changes into your life too.

As a Nutritional Therapist, highly trained in both western and Chinese dietetic principles, Elaine believes in a holistic approach to well-being through food, and she is committed to helping individuals and families around the world who want to be the best they can be with **'the 6 diet'**.

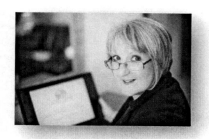

Her interest in combating diabetes is inherently personal. At the age of 13 Elaine lost her beloved grandmother who slipped into a diabetic coma and never regained consciousness: she was just 68 years old! Elaine remembers the pain:

"My gran was a mainstay in my life. I saw her every day. My school was just across the road, and she cooked my lunches instead of me staying for school dinners. The irony of her great desserts is not lost on me when I think about losing her to diabetes. When she died I was heartbroken, and I still feel the pain. With type 2 diabetes it's personal: it's my mission to combat this killer. The prevalence of type 2 diabetes is way out of control, and the stupid thing is that it doesn't have to be! All it takes is an understanding of how different foods affect your body, and how to eat to match your own unique needs. It's not just grandparents we have to worry about these days either: mums and dads and even the kids themselves are at much greater risk from type 2 diabetes than ever before. Together we can make it stop right now!"

Chapter 1:

Why blood-sugar control is vital

Introduction

So far, probably every 'diet' you have encountered is at least to some extent based on the notion of 'one-size-fits-all'. There is no other approach that I know of that really looks at *your* unique and individual needs, in terms of your health status, lifestyle factors, or true goals.

Maybe you have followed plans based on simplistic counting methods: counting calories / points / units etc. However, what these absolutely lack is a fundamental understanding that IT REALLY MATTERS WHAT THOSE CALORIES / POINTS / UNITS CONTAIN in terms of nutrient types and nutritional values. Your body has very different needs for carbohydrates, proteins and fats compared with other people. Indeed your own body has different needs for carbohydrates, proteins, fats etc. from one day to the next depending on what activities you will be undertaking. Surely this makes sense? It isn't something to understand only on a theoretical level — it is a hard fact that if you are sitting at a desk today your body has very different needs compared with tomorrow when you might be getting down to some serious housework or DIY, running around the park with the kids or working out, sightseeing etc.

Worse still are those diets totally based on another person's experience, remember that diets marketed by celebrities were created for that person alone — why should it work for you too? You don't have the same physical make up, genetics, medical history, lifestyle etc. as that person! You have your own unique biochemistry, so your diet needs to honour you and your own specific needs.

Most branded diet plans may appear to achieve a result but they WILL damage your health — and maybe you remember this being reported in the mainstream media as it became an increasingly recognised fact from about 2010. Unfortunately, I have seen first-hand the serious damage that some of my patients have incurred following fundamentally flawed diet and weight-loss regimes — but more about that in Chapter 2. And, nonetheless, there is still a lack of genuinely helpful and accurate information available to guide you to make better decisions.

'the 6 diet' delivers so much more than a diet and exercise programme — it provides you with all the education you need to understand your own body, your needs and the solutions that will help you to achieve your own goals.

To that end it is vital to spend some time really getting to know all about the unique, magical being that is YOU. **'the 6 diet'** is the start of a wonderful journey of discovery — getting to know yourself, your individual needs and the solutions to help you achieve your optimum body.

Let's start with some fundamentals about what your body will do with the different kinds of nutrients that you consume – how it will convert, use and store what it needs from the food that you provide to it.

Blood sugar balance is key

Most of us have heard the term 'blood sugar' often enough that we may think we know what it means: but we almost certainly take the term for granted. In reality, the blood sugar mechanism is complex, which is why it's so easy to get it drastically wrong. Its goal is to provide a steady supply of fuel to our cells around the clock.

We, like all animals, need to have a small amount of glucose available in our bloodstream all the time. Our brains require a small but constant supply of glucose otherwise they cannot function. If glucose levels fall too low, we experience confusion, shakiness – technically this is hypoglycaemia: a 'hypo'.

Glucose is the basic building block for energy. It fuels every bodily function that we have to perform, from those we control ourselves, such as walking, working, playing sport etc., to those that our own bodies take care of for us without us consciously being involved, for example breathing, making hormones, circulating our blood, maintaining our very ability to live!

We all need glucose, but we can have too much of this good thing! So let's explore a little about exactly what it is, how we get it, use it and store it. By really understanding some basic facts about glucose, you will discover why you could be eating good food but nonetheless storing excess body fat.

What is glucose?

Here comes a 'sciency bit'. If you don't like science please don't be put off, I've made it as quick and simple as I can to give you the knowledge you need. If you like science then great – here we go!

Glucose is a simple sugar: simple, that is, in respect of its molecular structure, $C_6H_{12}O_6$. The diagram showb is a representation of the chemical structure of glucose.

What makes it simple is that it is a small structure and contains only three common elements – carbon, hydrogen and oxygen. This very simple kind of sugar is called a *monosaccharide*.

We all need glucose, but surprisingly most of it doesn't come from actually eating it. Instead, most of our glucose needs are met by our digestive systems breaking down larger molecules of complex sugars and starch, known as carbohydrates. The very word carbohydrate is a mash up of the words carbon, hydrogen and oxygen – telling us exactly what it contains.

The time and digestive effort it takes for our bodies to convert other

$$H-C=O$$
$$H-C-OH$$
$$HO-C-H$$
$$H-C-OH$$
$$H-C-OH$$
$$CH_2OH$$

carbohydrates into glucose depends on the size and complexity of these larger molecules.

It will take very little time to convert another simple sugar into glucose. Let's take fructose as our first example. It is another monosaccharide, and it has exactly the same chemical formula as glucose, i.e. $C_6H_{12}O_6$. The only difference is that some of the elements are bonded together in a slightly different configuration. The diagram below shows the glucose and fructose molecules side -by-side. We could almost play 'spot-the-difference', they are so alike:

glucose   fructose

Because all the elements are present, in exactly the same amounts, and in a very similar structure, it takes very little time for the body to break apart the structure of fructose to reconfigure it as glucose. However, latest scientific thinking is that in reality this process takes place in the liver, and it is not a hugely efficient way to generate glucose. Very little of the fructose we eat actually ends up being converted to glucose. Instead the liver is more likely to turn it directly into certain kinds of fats: most often those linked with disease! This is why fructose is now being increasingly identified as a problem in our modern diet: high fructose sugars, especially high fructose corn syrup, is a staple part of many processed foods. Latest research studies are concluding that it's vital to restrict the amount of fructose sugars in our diet. In fact there are several monosaccharides all sharing the same formula, but with slightly different structures: allose, altrose, fructose, galactose, glucose, gulose, idose, mannose, sorbose, talose, tagatose. So many sugars – so little time to turn them into glucose! Fructose is the sugar found naturally in fruit, and as you can now see, some of the sugars from fruit can be used very quickly to provide glucose to the body. This is how it is possible to revive a diabetic patient rapidly with a small drink of orange juice! And yes – it's important to limit the amount of sugar we take in even from natural fresh fruit sources – especially fruit juices, but also whole fruits themselves!

Just for completeness I should mention that there are some monosaccharides that do not share their chemical formulae with glucose, but which still contain the basic building blocks of carbon, hydrogen and water.

The next most basic sugars are *disaccharides*. These contain two simple sugar molecules bonded together. Sucrose is one good example for us to use here – because it is basically just two sugar molecules, one fructose and the other glucose. Maltose is even better – it is simply two glucose molecules linked together. To convert maltose into glucose, all the digestive system has to do is break one bond from a molecule of maltose, and hey presto it has two molecules of glucose! So again, we can see that digesting disaccharides can generate glucose very quickly and easily.

More complicated carbohydrate structures contain longer chains of sugar molecules bound together. Where they have between two and ten individual sugar molecules in their structure they are called *ogliosaccharides*. The most complex, with even longer chains are the *polysaccharides*. The digestive system has to work harder, and it takes a little longer to break the chains, and reconfigure the elements to create glucose, but it still achieves this relatively quickly.

Complex sugars like those found in honey, syrups, milk etc., and the starches found in grains, potatoes, rice, beans and other carbohydrate-rich foods all contain chains of glucose that are bonded together with other substances. During digestion, enzymes break these bonds and release the glucose molecules which are then absorbed into your bloodstream.

Blood sugar balance

Blood sugar balance, or control, is the process of making sure we have enough, but not too much, glucose floating around in our bloodstreams at any one time. As we have already said, it is really vital that there is always some glucose there in the blood, to ensure our brains are able to function. Yet, the amount of glucose in our blood is never static. Our cells are constantly using up the glucose and burning it for energy. Replacing glucose that has been used up is essential for our brains. If the systems that regulate our blood sugar are healthy, the amount of glucose they provide is just enough to replace the glucose used! In this way, you could say we 'balance' our blood sugar.

Blood sugar levels naturally fluctuate throughout the day. However, there are two basic states that we need to consider. One is the fasting state and the other is the postprandial state.

The fasting state occurs when digestion has been completed, for example at night, while we sleep. With a reasonably balanced diet we enter the fasting state three hours after eating. In the fasting state our liver maintains normal blood sugar levels by releasing small amounts of glucose from the glycogen stores, or by converting protein into new glucose.

Our levels of insulin, which is a hormone released by the pancreas, tell our livers when they need to provide more glucose into the blood stream. When there is no new glucose being provided into the blood stream from digestion, little insulin is released and the low level alerts the liver to action.

We remain in the fasting state until we eat something. After eating, any pure glucose that was present in the food will be absorbed into our bloodstream usually within fifteen minutes. Just fifteen minutes? In fact if we eat glucose itself, it gets into our bloodstream and begins to feed our brain cells even before it leaves our mouth: again, think about how quickly a diabetic person can be revived with a glucose drink!

When we are talking about carbohydrates we usually think of two categories: refined and complex. Refined carbohydrates are those that will be converted into glucose within a few minutes, whereas complex carbohydrates will take a little longer.

Simple or refined carbohydrates, such as white flour or sugar, typically take between a half hour and an hour to provide glucose into our bloodstream. More complex carbohydrates, such as whole grains may take between one and three hours to be fully digested. During this so called postprandial state, the concentration of glucose in our blood will begin to rise as the glucose following digestion comes pouring in. For those of us with a healthy body, as soon as the glucose levels begin to rise, our pancreases are stimulated to deliver a large burst of insulin. Insulin's function is to activate receptors on our cell walls which allow these cells to take the circulating glucose molecules from our bloodstreams and either burn them for fuel or store them for future use. When insulin fails to activate these receptors a condition called 'insulin resistance' develops, eventually leading to full blown Type 2 Diabetes.

Whether or not we have healthy blood sugar systems, other nutrients also affect our blood sugar balance! Understanding how our bodies use and process different nutrient types and food groups helps us begin to see and understand why managing food intake is so vital to controlling energy, weight and shape.

Victims of our own evolutionary success?

Human bodies are highly effective glucose factories. We had to evolve that way or die out as a species – it's all down to our history.

Today we know that the great apes, including human beings first began to appear in Africa. Far from the famines we might now associate with that part of the world, in terms of food it was a very different place in prehistoric times. When the great apes began to emerge they flourished in a climate that served them an abundance of fruits – straight from the trees – all year round. They were essentially fruitarians – extracting the building blocks for energy directly from the sugars in which fruits are so naturally rich.

But then early man went walkabout, and strayed into areas of the world that couldn't support his fruit needs. He had to adapt or die. And gradually early man became adept at extracting glucose from any foods that he could find – by hunting or gathering.

As modern humans, we are brilliant at extracting our glucose needs very effectively and efficiently. To the extent that our dietary sugar needs are negligible, and our carbohydrate needs limited in order to support our normal, moderately active lifestyles. It isn't just that we don't need so much sugar or carbs. In our highly evolved state they can be quite simply harmful. Not so much unnecessary as dangerous!

Since sugar became a regular feature again in our diets – introduced back to us as a luxury commodity just a couple of hundred years ago - our consumption has continually risen. And it continues to rise. And with it the incidence and prevalence of obesity, diabetes and all its related concomitants are also rising – and killing us! We are most definitely victims of our evolutionary success – in danger of dying from too much sugar because our ancestors didn't die from a lack of it!

The deadly nature of sugar has been known for decades - but our consumption is now an addiction, and like any other addiction we are in its grip and we don't seem to be inclined to change that any time soon. Instead of burying our heads in the sand - or sweetie bag – it's time to educate ourselves. The key to finding the motivation to change is to fully understand the impact of our choices, to come face to face with the reality of what foods does – to heal and to harm us, and to have better information at out fingertips to help us make better food choices.

That education starts right here.

Getting the balance of carbohydrates, proteins and fats appropriate for *your* lifestyle

In very simple terms our bodies need two main things from food: they need energy, and they need a tool kit to develop, grow and repair our bodily tissues, and substances. The key to a great body is to balance these needs – and especially to make sure that the energy our bodies derive from food matches the amount of energy we need to fulfil our daily activities: too little energy spells trouble, too much often spells even more!

The Glycaemic Index (GI) is a measure of just how quickly a food will be converted into glucose, compared with glucose itself. The higher the GI, the faster the conversion process. So glucose itself scores a full 100 on the GI scale, with refined carbohydrates, made up of simple chains of sugars, scoring very highly, complex carbohydrates next, and protein and fats moderately or less. Our bodies can actually convert proteins into glucose, as we have seen, though the digestion process takes longer due to the complexity of protein structures.

Different mechanisms begin to kick in when we create more glucose than we need to meet our energetic needs. At first it isn't a huge issue. Through a process called glycolysis, the excess glucose is converted to glycogen which is stored in our livers and muscles. This is exactly what an athlete aims to do with so-called 'carb-loading': it's to make sure that as much glycogen as possible is stored, so that it can provide a back-up of energy for that long race! Glycogen is relatively quickly converted back into glucose, and subsequently energy, whenever we find ourselves in the situation of needing more energy than we have readily available. However, our glycogen stores are not endless – they do become full. On average we can store about 360 calories worth of energy in our glycogen stores – which means that if we need to draw upon our reserves for energy, we have 360 calories worth of activity before our bodies have to find a new source of nutrients to convert into glucose.

In situations where we digest carbohydrates without an immediate energy need AND our glycogen stores are full, yet another digestive process occurs. This time the excess glucose is converted into body fat, which is usually stored in close proximity to the liver – giving rise to the 'apple' shape or the 'muffin top'.

If we engage in physical activity and exhaust our readily available supplies of glucose, AND we empty our glycogen stores THEN our bodies turn to our fat stores for energy. When we develop a situation where our bodies begin to use fat for fuel our livers begin to transform protein into the glucose our brains need to keep going. If there is sufficient available the body will get this directly from the protein foods that we eat, such as meat or cheese. However, where there is insufficient dietary protein, our bodies will digest our own muscle tissues.

Let's think about this really closely for a moment: when our bodies begin to burn off our body fat for energy, our livers also begin to break down our lean tissues? Yes!

Because our body can 'eat' our own muscle tissues in this way, inappropriate diets that are too low in protein result in a dangerous loss of them. This is one of the ways that most branded diet plans are fundamentally flawed and will lead to unhealthy consequences!

So called 'healthy' food products tend to be reduced or low in fat. The diet industry has relied on low fat alternatives for many years, and there is no sign that this is about to change any day now! Yet, a close look at the product labels is revealing... take out fat, and something has to replace it. Usually this is sugar! These foods have a manufactured imbalance of carbohydrates, proteins and fats, which together are called the 'macronutrients'. Low-sugar or sugar-free food products, which essentially seek to eliminate the most highly refined carbohydrates, are no solution either! You can be sure that any dietary regime that requires you to eliminate or seriously reduce any of the macronutrients is fundamentally flawed: for health and well-being you absolutely need all three regularly. Losing weight like this rarely involves losing just fat! Your healthy tissues may well begin to suffer too – and if that damage is not addressed then poor health is a genuine risk.

Proteins and fats are primarily needed to provide the components of the tool kit required for bodily development, growth and repair. They are complex molecules which require a lot of digestive effort, and are converted much more slowly than carbohydrates. When consumed together with carbohydrates they also slow down the rate at which the carbohydrates can be digested – because the digestive system has to work on the meal as a whole. This is the basis of Glycaemic Load (GL). We can even out the rate at which our bodies can convert food into available energy by combining carbohydrates with other nutrients to make a meal that is converted to energy at a rate we can use it, depending on our activities at that time of course. The lower the GL of a meal, the more steadily our digestion will function to derive energy from the food, which means our glycogen stores are not always crammed full, and we will be protected from depositing the abdominal fat that gives us that characteristic apple shape or muffin-top.

There is much more to say about proteins and fats later – and we will come back to them again.

With a little knowledge and **'the 6 diet'**, you can eat to meet your own energetic requirements, whilst protecting, and even improving your muscles and other tissues, benefiting your figure and health and emotional well-being at the same time.

The consequences of poor blood sugar balance

Here's what happens when our blood sugar is not properly balanced.

As we have now discovered, when our brains detect too much glucose in the blood stream, as a result of digesting food, our pancreases secrete insulin to help the transportation of glucose into the cells for metabolism, or for conversion to glycogen or fat. Consequently, this causes a dip in blood-sugar. When our brains detect such a dip, they prompt our bodies to call for food: hence we feel hungry.

The more we can even out the dips in blood-sugar, the more comfortable we are, feeling satisfied or fuller for longer. This is our ideal situation. It is created by eating foods that will deliver a low GL meal, causing the rate of food conversion to provide a steady release of glucose. It means that our food provides a supply of energy at the same rate we need it, until eventually it is used up. Our bodies then invoke their hunger response, prompting us to eat again to maintain the glucose / energy supply.

When we consume high GI foods or high GL meals that generate glucose very quickly, at a pace much faster than our bodies require energy, we secrete insulin in large quantities, and fast! Having too much glucose in our blood streams isn't a good thing! For now, picture this: we eat a meal rich in refined carbohydrates, our blood is saturated with glucose, we secrete lots of insulin to remove the excess glucose which is converted to glycogen or fat. Our blood-sugar dips again very quickly, and we are hungry again in no time at all.

We easily find ourselves in a cycle of binging and rapid hungering, needing to eat again very quickly. In fact our bodies never seem to be satisfied and because we become accustomed to needing more glucose, it tends to be those very sweet foods that our bodies crave.

So the very best we can hope to experience if we don't eat to control our blood sugar levels is frequent hunger, food cravings, especially for sweet and sugary foods, and the resultant apple-shape or muffin top!

Sadly, the story doesn't end at that!

When we have low-blood sugar – either on-going or as a result of some of the lows experienced as a result of large fluctuations – our bodies will conserve as much glucose as they can for our brains. This means that other parts of our bodies may be deprived until another source of glucose can be found – either from eating, or as a result of our livers releasing some from glycogen or from fat stores. We may experience energy dips, especially mid-morning or mid-afternoon. We may also experience general tiredness, fatigue, confusion and an inability to concentrate, irritability, an inability to communicate well, or even 'the shakes'. Many cases of insomnia, particularly characterised by waking in the middle of the night, are due to low blood sugar – causing us to wake. Even though we don't always recognise the reason or take appropriate action, it is a prompt for us to feed our bodies again.

When we continue to eat sugars and refined carbohydrates or high GI foods, our bodies have to secrete lots and lots of insulin, too much and too often. The healthy process as we have described above, in which insulin helps our cells to absorb the glucose through the cell walls, begins to break down. The cell walls no longer respond to the insulin, and the glucose remains in the blood stream at too high levels.

This is called 'insulin resistance', and it is effectively our inability to process glucose properly. This condition has different names, depending on where in the world you live. You may have heard it called 'Metabolic Syndrome'? Or 'Syndrome X'? Cardiometabolic Syndrome? Reaven's Syndrome? Or in Australia you may know it as CHAOS, which is a brilliantly descriptive name for its consequences!

Insulin resistance is essentially a combination of medical disorders that, when occurring together, increase the risk of developing cardiovascular diseases, strokes and diabetes. It is associated with high levels of triglycerides (a type of fat) in the blood stream, cholesterol problems, and high blood pressure. It is not to be taken at all lightly: in general, someone having insulin resistance is twice as likely to develop heart disease and five times as likely to develop diabetes as someone with normal insulin function.

Insulin is not the only hormone that responds badly to too much sugar

Most people are not aware that a hormone called leptin plays an enormous role in the development of obesity. In fact, it's only recently that scientists themselves have properly begun to understand the role of leptin.

Leptin, crucially, is a hormone that is just as important as insulin in determining your risk for type 2 diabetes and other serious diseases. Its job is to regulate our hunger – essentially it tells us when we are full, and to stop eating. However, as with insulin, we can become insensitive to the effects of leptin, and resistant to its messages. When this occurs we are more likely to store our fat around our organs and abdomen: more visceral fat!

So here's how it goes:

- We eat a diet that contains too many sugars and other carbohydrates, typically from grains which our bodies convert to sugar very quickly
- When we don't need the sugar for energy, it is stored as body fat
- This activity in turn causes a surge in leptin
- When we are constantly producing leptin our bodies become resistant to leptin just as it can become insulin-resistant and no longer hear its own signals to stop eating, burn fat, or pass up sugary foods.
- The result? We stay hungry, we crave sweets, and our bodies store ever more fat.
- When our bodies routinely store this much excess visceral fat, we increase our risk of ill health, including developing type 2 diabetes!

Introducing a question of inflammation?

The most recent research shows us that type 2 diabetes is essentially an inflammatory disease. We know that not everyone who develops type 2 diabetes is obese and not everyone who is obese develops type 2 diabetes. Doctors are starting to refer to the latter group as 'healthy obese'. So just what is the common thread linking those who do go on to develop type 2 diabetes? It's inflammation! Which foods are linked with causing the greatest level of inflammation? That's right – it's sugar and refined carbohydrate foods. The reason why sugar is so incredibly damaging to our modern human bodies is becoming much clearer to scientists. Yet the food and diet industries at large are showing no signs of adapting their own claims for so-called 'healthy' foods. More low-fat, high sugar/carb products find their way onto our supermarket shelves at an alarming rate – shockingly still labelled as the 'healthy' choice.

Worse is that mainstream dietary advice for diabetes, promoted by the NHS in the UK, advises that between 40% and 60% of our diet should be made up of grains and starches. Our healthcare professionals are only just waking up to the fact that their advice doesn't work: well the statistics speak loud and clear! Reviewing their own current advice is still only a plan within the NHS, however, so don't expect it to change in the immediate future.

Further, as I write, DiabetesUK, defying logic and research findings, clearly declare on their website that sugar consumption does not lead to type 2 diabetes!

There is little wonder that so many people still don't understand the dangers hidden in their dietary choices. Thankfully, you have found **'the 6 diet'**, and all the latest, most scientifically up-to-date, information you need to point you towards a healthier you!

The roles of proteins and fats

Consuming proteins and fats is not simply a way of lowering the GL value of a meal to assist with our blood sugar control. Really that is a minor role for them in terms of our overall health and well-being. They are equally as important as carbohydrates, having vital functions of their own. We look much more closely at these vital nutrients in Chapter 3.

Chapter 2:

Body Composition

The problem with most diets?

So the question is this: if you plan to change your eating habits to achieve your very best body and health, what is the baseline against which you will measure your progress and, ultimately, success?

Whilst you may know your weight, do you know what your weight comprises? Is it fat? Lean tissue? Cell mass? Water? And how healthy are you? Do your cells function properly? Are nutrients readily absorbed into your body? Are toxic waste products efficiently removed from your cells? Does the amount of water in your body constitute healthy hydration or water retention? Does your chronological age match your biological age?

HAVE YOU INADVERTANTLY CAUSED DAMAGE TO YOUR MUSCLES OR OTHER TISSUES BY INAPPROPRIATE DIETING?

Is the idea that losing weight may be harmful new to you? It's a topic that began to hit our mainstream press between 2009 and 2012, when it was reported that yo-yo dieting, serially losing and gaining weight, could be harmful to your health. More harmful than staying fat! How can that be?

The disturbing truth is this - most weight loss diets encourage your body to sacrifice healthy lean tissue rather than body fat. This is illustrated wonderfully by some clinical research carried out in Denmark. The researchers looked at men and women on a variety of well-known slimming diet approaches. On average the weight lost by men comprised 41% healthy lean tissue. For women the lean tissue equated to 35% of the total weight lost. Here you might be forgiven for thinking that women fare better than men – but when you take into equation the fact that men carry a greater percentage of lean tissue than women you can see that is not the case. This is further highlighted by the findings about what happens when weight is regained. The same Danish team discovered that on regaining weight the lean tissue is not restored: of the weight regained by men only 24% was lean tissue, and by women a mere 15%! This means that serially losing and regaining weight eventually replaces healthy lean tissues by body fat.

Healthy lean tissues and body fat have very different functions in the body, and behave very differently. In terms of using energy derived from the food you eat, it is only the lean tissue that burns calories. Fat is simply a storehouse of those calories. Remember we talked in Chapter 1 about body fat being stored as a result of excess glucose not immediately needed for energy? This means that if you end a diet with proportionally more fat – having sacrificed some calorie-burning lean tissue - your body can make use of fewer calories before you begin to store more body fat. You are never in a position to go back to eating the way you did before the weight loss diet because you can eat fewer calories after the diet than before the diet before you start to regain weight – *easy fast weight regain = next diet, and so the yo-yoing continues!*

It is absolutely vital that any weight loss diet focuses on helping you to lose body fat rather than lean tissue – but sadly most weight loss approaches fail to recognise this importance.

A common measure associated with diet, weight loss, and health is Body Mass Index (BMI). This has been used for a long time as an indicator of whether or not we are a 'healthy' weight for our height. It still governs so much of the thinking not only within the healthcare services, but also the diet industry. However, it is acknowledged to be a flawed measure. Flawed because it takes no account whatsoever of your bodily make-up. You can have a fabulously toned and muscular body yet be declared 'obese' according to the BMI measure. Conversely, you can be light, but predominantly composed of fatty tissue, yet be considered to be an appropriate weight and therefore by association thought to be healthy. Yet we know, of course, that the muscular person is the one much more likely to enjoy good health, a great quality of life and longevity!

Other measures such as calliper tests, hip/waist ratios etc. will readily tell you about the state of the outside of your body, but they will tell you very little, at best, about what is going on beneath your skin. Fundamentally these tests tell you little more than what you can readily judge by looking in the mirror or from the fit of your clothes – are you enjoying your ideal body image?

And what about your health?

It's time to introduce you to your BODY COMPOSITION.

Body composition

This may be new terminology, or a perhaps a new concept for you. If so, then here is some crucial new learning for you! If you are lucky enough to already be familiar with the concept, then here is some crucial revision for you! Either way, here is a list of questions that will be really useful for you – they are key to helping you meet your combined goals of a great looking body and achieving optimum health!

What is body composition?

'Body Composition' is essentially the technical term used to describe the balance of the different components that make up our bodies. At the most simplistic level, some people in the diet and fitness industry consider it to be a measure of the relative ratios of fat mass to fat-free mass. If you investigate this further you will find that others expand on that to include muscle, bone, organs and other bodily tissues. A medical dictionary definition breaks this down further into the relative proportions of protein, fat, water, and mineral components in the body.

'the 6 diet' considers a more sophisticated view of body composition: we'll define it as the balance of your bio-chemical make-up, in terms of:

- Fat, which is made up of:
    o Essential fats / lipids
    o Non-essential fats
    o Water
- Fat-free mass – which comprises:
    o Muscle
    o Bone
    o Organs
    o Tissues

It's also essential for us to recognise that muscle, bone, organs and other tissues are all made up of specialised cells, and that they are in turn made up of proteins/amino acids, fats/lipids, minerals/trace elements and water.

Why is it important to think of body composition to this level of detail? Well, our bodies require nutritional support for all these things – and if we don't properly understand these building blocks, then we won't properly understand how to nourish ourselves properly, or to provide all the tools our bodies need to develop, maintain, repair themselves.

How individual is my body composition?

The short answer is 'totally'! You can be assured that *your* body composition is *yours alone*. Think of all the things that make you totally unique: no one else shares your finger prints, the patterns and colours in your eyes, your dental imprints, DNA or genetic make-up etc. These are all things that can be used to very accurately identify you and you alone, and they are related to your own unique body composition.

Now, for sure there are some averages that can be used as guidelines to suggest whether you have a healthy or unhealthy body composition. These tend to be based on standard reference values according to age and gender – which is to say that healthy men and women, boys and girls tend to have body composition values within certain ranges. However, these can only ever be guidelines.

So my size and shape depends on my body composition?

Absolutely!

You will have noticed how different individuals of about the same height and weight (and therefore BMI) may have very different body shapes. This is because muscle tissue takes up less space in our bodies than fat tissue. So, for sure your body composition, as well as your weight, determines your overall size. The density of your bodily tissues and the amount of body fat that you carry are key factors in determining your overall outward appearance in terms of size.

Shape largely depends on the relative distributions of fat in various parts of the body. Typically we may think of the so called 'apple' and 'pear' shapes – where fat is primarily focused around the abdomen or hips, bottoms and thighs respectively. Also, we may think of some people, usually women, as being 'top heavy' having large breasts, which are predominantly comprised of fatty tissue, or shoulders and upper arms etc. Overall shape is again completely governed by body composition.

There are three types of body shape, or 'somatotypes': these being ectomorphs, mesomorphs and endomorphs. People with an ectomorphic body shape have characteristically long and thin muscles and limbs. They have a low capacity for storing body fat or for building muscle, and therefore are generally slim. Mesomorphs are generally characterised by medium bones, a solid torso, and low levels of body fat. They tend to have wide shoulders with a narrow waist, and are usually referred to as muscular, being predisposed to build muscle but not store fat. Endomorphs are characterised by a predisposition to store excess body fat, and typically have a wide waist and a large bone structure.

However, what you see in the mirror, in terms of your overall shape, is only a part of the body composition story. Your reflection can only tell you something about the amount of fat that your body deposits on the outside, just below your skin – this is called adipose tissue – and where it is primarily located. It gives you a picture of your body size and shape, but nothing useful about your overall health. This is partly because fat can also be deposited inside the body where it is not necessarily obvious – around, or even inside, your internal organs for example. Fat deposited around the organs is called 'visceral' fat and we'll come back to that a little later.

How does water affect my body?

Water is a crucial body component BUT people can be naively simplistic about water in respect of body composition. How much water we hold in our bodies is one factor – we already know that we need to be well hydrated. Water generally represents 45% to 60% of an adult's total body weight. Women tend to have less than men, because generally a healthy woman will carry more body fat than a healthy male and we all carry more water in muscle than we do in fat. Approximately 80% of muscle tissue is made up of water, while only 20% of body fat is comprised of water. This explains the fact that muscle weighs more than fat! It's because lipids are lighter than water - think of how the grease floats on top of the water when you are washing the dishes!

The overall amount of water in our bodies, however, is only half the story. A second crucial factor, when thinking about how water affects the body, is WHERE the water is located. We really need water to be held inside the cells in our bodies: this is true hydration. Water held outside of the boundary created by the cell walls is merely water retention. If you've experienced water retention you will know how uncomfortable and bloating this phenomenon can be!

So, when thinking about body composition, it is not enough to know just the percentage of water in your body – you really need to know that you are hydrated rather than retaining water. Proper hydration is necessary because water plays a vital role in all our bodily processes, bio-chemical reactions, lubrication, nutrient delivery, waste disposal, heat dispersion and temperature regulation. Even slight levels of dehydration can play havoc with some of our bodily functions: it can lead to anything from dizziness or confusion, to coma or even death.

Is my body composition related to how much I need to eat?

Indeed!

Our lean bodily tissue, or fat-free mass, needs fuel in order to function. Our fatty tissue, or fat mass, doesn't – it is primarily a store of fuel. Muscles, organs, and other lean tissues are described as 'metabolically active'. This means that the more lean mass we have compared to fat mass, the more fuel our bodies need to function. The higher the ratio between fat-free mass and fat mass, the higher our metabolic rate. So, a muscular person <u>needs</u> more food to maintain their bodily functions than someone carrying an excess of body fat! How great is that?

Our bodies also need to function effectively even when we are asleep, and therefore have a fuel requirement whether or not we are active. The amount of energy that we need to derive from our food, without taking into account any of our daily activities is called the Basal Metabolic Rate (BMR).

So – knowing your individual body composition helps you to determine how much food is appropriate uniquely for you by providing you with a very accurate measure of your BMR. Of course, the more active you are in your daily life the more fuel your body requires to serve your activities. So, to calculate exactly how much fuel, measured in calories, you need to consume on a daily basis you need to take into account your BMR and activity levels.

Food packaging typically estimates that an adult women needs to consume 2000 calories per. day, and an adult man, 2500 calories per. day. It's highly unlikely for your body composition, and BMR, to correspond with an average taken across an entire population; you will clearly see the pitfalls in such generalised nutritional, dietary and lifestyle advice. This is why you need an individually tailored programme to meet your own needs, and deliver your own goals for your best shape, weight, size and state of optimum health! Following a programme created for someone else won't necessarily deliver the same great benefits for you!

Does my body composition relate to my health?

Yes, and to a VERY large extent!

Expert scientists at Cambridge University in England recognise the importance of body composition in how it relates to health:

"It is important when studying obesity to be able to measure body composition, [it is] a useful measure for predicting health."

At the simplest level, we know that obesity and being over-weight is linked with serious illnesses such as diabetes, heart disease and some types of cancer.

We all need some body fat for overall health. It helps to protect our internal organs, provides energy and regulates hormones which are important for a wide range of bodily functions. It also stores some vitamins, so when we consume more than we need they are not lost through our normal waste disposal mechanisms.

Too little body fat, therefore, can also be detrimental to our health.

It is too simplistic, however, to relate health to the overall amount of body fat. Where it is stored is also a key to your health. As we have previously discussed, an excess of fat around the abdominal organs, known as visceral fat, is associated with risk factors such as insulin resistance, diabetes and high blood pressure and it can be a useful measure for predicting health. Research has now identified the dangers associated with visceral fat. Fundamentally it is because these fat cells behave quite differently from subcutaneous fat, the kind stored just below our skins. We have more subcutaneous fat cells than we have visceral fat cells, but the visceral fat cells become bigger. When subcutaneous fat cells become 'full', our bodies create more – not great because once your body has generated more fat cells they don't reduce in number again. Visceral fat cells, on the other hand, keep growing until they finally disintegrate, a process technically called 'apoptosis'. At this point they produce inflammatory molecules, called cytokines, that are then circulated via the blood stream, with the potential to cause inflammation anywhere in the body. Cytokines are thought to be responsible for hardening of the arteries, heart disease, high blood pressure, high cholesterol, some types of cancers and tumours, strokes, sleep apnoea, some degenerative diseases, depressions, osteoporosis in women, and yes, type 2 diabetes. Again here is the link between diabetes and inflammation!

This inflammation continues – becoming a permanent state. It is a chronic condition—constantly happening, again and again.

So, how much visceral fat is too much? After all, we need some visceral fat to cushion our organs. But many of us have far too much of it. Men are at high risk if they have a waistline of 40 inches or greater whereas for women the limit is 35 inches. Once you hit that limit it's already too late - you're probably already in a perpetually inflamed state.

But does that mean we can't do anything about it? The first thing you must understand is that there is absolutely NO quick fix solution. No fast weight-loss diet will help; no gimmicky pills or exercise gadgets will help; no gastric band surgery or liposuction procedure will touch visceral fat. Only a sensible, gradual, packed full of appropriate nutrition approach to food for life will do the trick. I call it **'the 6 diet'**! It can efficiently and effectively help you to reduce your abdominal fat specifically – bringing you back to levels below risk. The sooner you catch it the better!

And here's a rather curious fact: it isn't only obviously fat people who can suffer a build-up of visceral fat. Thin people can get it too. It's a phenomenon that has its own acronym: TOFI. That's 'thin on the outside, fat on the inside'. And it is linked with a sedentary lifestyle in which we don't burn off all the energy generated from our consumption of carbohydrates. Next time your thin friend tells you they can eat anything they like and get away with it, gently tell them about TOFI – you could be doing them a huge favour, because unless they address the problem, just like their overweight counterparts, they too are at risk of all the same health problems.

Fat stored within organs is also problematic e.g. fat stored in the liver is called 'liver steatosis', or more commonly 'fatty liver syndrome'.

We get a clearer picture of how body composition and health are related if we take a closer look right down to a cellular level. Here's why:

Every cell in your body has a membrane separating the inside of the cell from its external environment. Nutrients from food need to be able to pass through the cell wall to enable the internal parts of the cell to do their specialised jobs. After that, waste products need to be passed out again so they can removed. The technical term for this is 'cell metabolism'. It is too simplistic to think of the cell wall in the same way that we might think of a balloon – simply a barrier between the outside and the inside of the cell. It is a highly intelligent part of our bodies, and is largely made of lipid / fat. This is another reason why the location of fats in your body plays a crucial role in determining your health. If the cell wall is not able to function, then the cell cannot function, and really serious illnesses begin to develop. Consider this: every major illness involves the inability of a group of specialised cells to carry out their normal function, e.g. cancer cells are mutant cells, degenerative diseases involve a breakdown of cell structures so they cannot function normally. Here we have another potential link with diabetes: in type 2 diabetes, as we have already seen, the pancreas can usually secrete sufficient insulin, but the cells become insensitive to the presence of that insulin, and fail to allow glucose to pass through the cell wall into the cell itself where it can be metabolised.

One of the measures that can be derived from knowing your body composition is something called your 'phase angle'. Simply, it is a measure that shows how well the walls of the cells are functioning, being a measure of their integrity. Phase angle is nothing new in the medical world; it has featured for decades as a way to predict the prognosis in people who develop serious illnesses. As a result, standard ranges for phase angle have also been devised according to gender and age. There is a lot to follow later about what your phase angle means to you!

But for now, it is suffice to say that people with optimal body composition are typically healthier, move more easily and efficiently, and in general, feel better than those with less-than-ideal body composition. Achieving a more optimal body composition goes a long way toward improving your quality of life and overall wellness.

So my body composition affects my overall quality of life?

When you understand how your body composition affects your health, it takes only a small amount of imagination to see how it also affects your overall quality of life.

People with poor health often have a correspondingly poor quality of life. Pain, immobility, poor respiratory function, heart disease, low immunity, inflammatory illnesses, skin problems – the list goes on! All affect how well we can join in with our families and friends and enjoy normal daily activities. The side effects of medication to treat illness can also be debilitating.

If you haven't yet developed diabetes, serious health considerations may seem very distant right now. You may be lucky enough to have escaped such illness yet, but failure to take your body composition into account may be a ticking bomb preparing to detonate in your future! Of course, if you are already diabetic you are now faced with this reality. You can use this as motivation to improve your own body composition!

So let's look at some other common everyday issues. Consider how your overall body image and confidence affect your daily life. Your appearance is an outward manifestation of your body composition. At the most obvious end of this spectrum is your shape and size. But also think about your complexion, skin, hair, nails etc. Are you embarrassed by your body in any way? Does it prevent you or inhibit you from joining in and enjoying a wide range of pleasurable activities? What about your mood and emotional wellbeing? Are you really making the most of your life?

Yes, it's true, you really cannot separate any of these issues from your body composition. Because every bodily function, including your *mental and emotional functions*, depends on the efficiency of your body at that cellular level, your ability to enjoy life physically, energetically and in every way is so closely wrapped up in your body composition. Your outward appearance, physical health, and inner sense of wellbeing are all potentially affected by your body composition!

Does my body composition influence my longevity?

Here is where you need to know more about your phase angle! As we've said, phase angle is a measure that has been used for a long time in medicine to predict the outcomes for people suffering from serious illness. Of course, in saying that I alluded to the notion that your phase angle is a general indication of how well your body is functioning overall.

Just as there are standard reference values for other aspects of body composition according to age and gender, there are similar values for phase angle. Typically men have greater phase angles than women –

the higher the value generally the more athletic you are considered to be. Also, in terms of age our phase angles typically peak in our twenties, and decline quite sharply in our seventies and eighties.

'the 6 diet' tells you therefore, that you can judge your body performance against others in your own and different age groups.

In the introduction to this book it was explained that most diet plans WILL adversely affect health. In terms of phase angle it is not untypical, in my own clinical experience, to see men and women, having followed ill-advised dietary regimes for a period of time, achieving measures relating to age categories twenty or even thirty years greater than their own actual age. In short – their biological age is measured at twenty to thirty years older than their chronological age!

Shocked? Me too. I never cease to despair at what people unwittingly do to themselves by faithfully trying to do the right thing, but with the wrong advice!

This is where **'the 6 diet'** is genuinely different.

By not only understanding these issues, and promoting better messages, but by seeking to impart them to you too, we want to help you on your journey towards a longer, healthier and more fulfilled life! You can use **'the 6 diet'** to be the very best version of you!

So can I improve my body composition?

Absolutely!

Depending on your starting point, it should take about 12 weeks to see tangible improvements IF you are prepared to make the necessary changes:

- Your body shape will change
- You may lose some weight (but remember – muscle weighs more than fat so as your body composition changes and you swap fat for muscle your weight itself may not be your best measure of change!)
- You will feel more energetic – tiredness and fatigue will begin to fade away
- Your complexion will begin to look more glowing
- Any symptoms that you experience now may begin to improve
- You will have an increased inner sense of well-being
- You will feel more confident in yourself
- You will make better dietary choices, benefiting yourself and your loved ones

- Your balance of fat mass to fat-free mass will improve
- Your body's ability to hydrate instead of retain water will improve
- Your biological age will begin to align with your chronological age (it may even undertake it!)
- Your overall quality of life will improve

Let's look at Anne's case. She presented in my clinic in August 2013 as follows:

> Anne was diagnosed as 'pre-diabetic'. She was showing all the signs of insulin resistance and her blood glucose levels were beginning to rise. Her body composition was curious: though Anne weighed only 9½ stones she had a disproportionate amount of abdominal fat. Her body composition test showed that of her total body weight 40% was made up of body fat, and she had a waist measurement of 36 inches. It was crucial for Anne to lose that abdominal fat without sacrificing any of her already insufficient lean tissue. I created a personalised dietary plan for her, using all the principles of **'the 6 diet'**, and closely monitored Anne's progress – regularly carrying out body composition tests to ensure that her results were beneficial.
>
> Both Anne and I have been delighted by her progress: after just 4 weeks she had lost 4lbs in weight, but 5lbs in body fat! Using appropriate nutrition her body had converted 1lb of body fat into lean healthy tissue! Her waist measurement had already reduced by 2 inches. She is the proof that using correct nutritional principles you can massively improve body composition and body shape in a very short time.
>
> Ultimately Anne is no longer considered at risk of type 2 diabetes, and her doctor has no reason to prescribe medications to reduce Anne's blood sugar levels.

Here's the rub: **'the 6 diet'** advice can only work for you if you actually follow it! You are going to get great advice here, but now that you are aware of the importance of your body composition the responsibility for looking after it is all yours!

How can I determine my body composition?

There are several different kinds and levels of test. Whichever you choose may depend on the availability in your area, and, indeed, your budget?

Simple tests

BMI

Whilst BMI is not really adequate, if you know that you are carrying excess body fat then it is at least a starting point. If you have a muscular body it really isn't going to be your best guide!

You can calculate your BMI using a relatively straight forward formula:

- Measure your height in metres
- Measure your weight in kilograms
- Calculate: $\dfrac{\text{your weight in kilograms}}{(\text{your height in metres})^2}$

So, for example, if your height is 1.65 metres (about 5 feet and 5 inches), and you weigh 76 kilograms (about 12 stones), your BMI is calculated as: $\dfrac{76}{1.65^2}$

This gives a BMI score of 28. So what does this mean?

In the west a BMI ranging between 19 and 25 is considered to be a good weight; 26-30 indicates overweight; 30-40 is considered to indicate obesity; 40+ corresponds with morbid obesity. However, whilst this is generally considered appropriate for people of Caucasian origins, it is questionable as an indicator for people of some Asian origins because they typically have smaller frame sizes. The health problems that we associate with overweight and obese measures in the west are often seen to occur at lower BMI measures for some people of Chinese, Malaysian and Indian origins. Clinical research, therefore, suggests that significant risks are posed in these populations for individuals in the BMI range of 22-24, and that serious risks occur in the BMI range 25-27.

Again, this is a great example of why those 'one-size-fits-all' plans are inadequate to ensure we all get the great results they invariably promise.

Waist to Hip Ratio

The purpose of this test is to determine the ratio of the waist circumference to the hip circumference, and has been shown to provide an indication of the likelihood or risk of developing coronary heart disease.

It requires only a simple calculation of the measurement of the waist girth divided by the measurement of the hip girth. This can be done in inches or centimetres.

The table below gives general guidelines for acceptable levels for hip to waist ratio.

	Healthy		At risk		
	Excellent	Good	Average	High	Extreme
Male	< 0.85	0.85 – 0.90	0.90 – 0.95	0.95 – 1.00	> 1.00
Female	< 0.75	0.75 – 0.80	0.80 – 0.85	0.85 – 0.90	> 0.90

Calliper test

This test involves pinching the skin to measure the thickness of the skin folds. This is done at 4 defined locations on your body: on the upper arm, at the back or underneath side near to the triceps muscle; on the upper arm, at the front over the biceps muscle; on the back just below the shoulder blade; and at the waistline.

You will need specialist callipers, which should come with their own instruction manual depending on the type that you buy.

The purpose of the test is to assess the total amount of fat on your body. It is also possible to estimate your total percent of body fat.

More sophisticated tests

Bioelectrical impedance analysis (BIA)

This test measures body composition by sending a small electrical signal through the body. The amount of resistance encountered by the signal is indicative of the type of tissue that it is passing through, e.g. fat, muscle, bone, water etc.

There is a wide variety of machines, ranging from those that look like bathroom scales, to more complex machines that operate in the same way as ECGs, using sticky pads located at specific points on the body which are then connected by electrodes to the measuring device itself.

The latter is the kind that I personally favour and use in my own clinical practice, as it is easily portable yet gives a good degree of accuracy across a wide range of results, including fat mass, fat-free mass, cell mass, bone mass, amounts and percentages of water – indicating hydration v. water retention, BMR, BMI and phase angle.

Dual Energy X-ray Absorptiometry (DEXA)

This test involves the use of a type of X-ray machine that measures overall body fat, regional fat, lean mass and bone density. It is used increasingly for a variety of clinical and research applications. Total body or estimated total body scans using DEXA give accurate and precise measurements including bone mineral content (BMC), bone mineral density (BMD), lean tissue mass, fat tissue mass etc.

These measurements are extremely replicable, making them excellent for monitoring pharmaceutical therapy, nutritional or exercise intervention, sports training or other body composition altering programs. They are also fast, simple, non-invasive, and claim to expose the subject to only low levels of radiation (though I would say that ANY exposure to radiation needs careful consideration).

Ultrasonagraphy (US)

This technique uses sound waves to visualise structures in the body. It is used to measure the amount of fat in the midriff (abdomen) of volunteers. In particular it measures visceral fat (the fat around abdominal organs) and subcutaneous fat (the fat under the skin) and liver steatosis (fat within the liver). By using multiple points a measurement of body composition can be made. Ultrasound has the advantage of being able to also directly measure muscle thickness and quantify intramuscular fat.

Air Displacement Plethysmography (ADP)

This technique uses air to measure body composition. The subject enters a sealed chamber, usually egg-shaped, that measures their body volume through the displacement of air in the chamber. Body volume is combined with body weight (mass) in order to determine body density. The technique then estimates the percentage of body fat and lean body mass (LBM) through mathematical equations (for the density of fat and fat free mass).

Magnetic Resonance Imaging (MRI) and Computed Tomography (CT) scans

MRI and CT scans give the most precise body composition measures to-date. Many pharmaceutical companies are therefore very interested in this procedure to estimate body composition measures before and after drug therapy especially in drugs that might change body composition. They are very specialist, and extremely expensive, so it's highly unlikely that you'll be able to benefit from them without a real medical need. However, I thought I would mention it – at least to press home the point that body composition is something to be taken very seriously.

How can I change my body composition?

Well, I guess that is exactly what the rest of this book is about!

We'll specifically look at all the factors that may influence your body composition, identify some of the things that will be detrimental, and propose the solutions. Of course, your dietary regime is going to play a huge part in your transformation, and **'the 6 diet'** takes into account your individuality. No 'one-size-fits-all' approach is good enough for you or for **'the 6 diet'**!

Is there anything that might limit how much my body composition will change?

Yes, there are several factors that might mitigate how much you will be able to change your body composition.

You may be familiar with the idea that your genetic make-up determines almost everything about you? You may be surprised to learn that this is only true to a certain extent? Apart from diseases and illnesses that are caused by actual chromosomal abnormalities – things like Down's Syndrome, Haemophilia, Huntington's Chorea and others - you are not as hostage to your gene pool as you may think.

Rather than dictating the course of your life, your genes are mere potentialities. They may trigger certain conditions, but ONLY IF they are able to be expressed. They may be little booby traps waiting to trip you up, but if you tread carefully you absolutely can avoid their consequences! For example, people with a cancer gene are not necessarily doomed to develop this horrible disease, nor are those with the so-called 'obesity gene' destined to be obese! The more you understand yourself, the more you respect and properly nurture yourself, the more you can defy your negative genes!

You may not be able to fully combat their effects, especially in terms of inherited body shapes etc., but you certainly don't have to be defeated by them. Your genes are not your excuse to accept or expect less of yourself!

What you may find more surprising is the crucial effect that your experience in the womb has on your body composition at birth, and potentially throughout your life. Your mother's nutrition, health and emotional well-being during her pregnancy did have a definite influence on your body composition. Of course, it may be a little late for you to change this for yourself, but prospective mums might be interested to know this on behalf of their own children!

Your age may be a defining factor – as I have already said, all of our body compositions naturally change as we age. However, that is not to say that you cannot make some very real and beneficial changes starting right now! Your biological age can easily become less than your chronological age!

Your current health status right now is important. If serious illness has already developed, it may not be possible to put Pandora back into her box. That said, having tested some patients within my clinical practice, and even after serious illness, including cancer, I am delighted that they have been able to carefully manage their way back to a body composition considered to be healthy, or even better than standard, for their gender and age!

Most of all your success depends on you! If you have a positive attitude towards yourself, and indeed to the idea of change, then the sky is possibly your limit. Just give yourself 12 weeks of real committed effort on **'the 6 diet'**, and see what you will accomplish.

Chapter 3:

Nutrition

Nutritional basics

You might have been led to believe that our modern understanding of nutrition is complete. After all the food and diet industries have adhered to the same advice for decades now. We have been led to understand that low-fat is key to weight loss and good health, and, simplistically, that sugar and salt aren't that great either! The low fat message is one that continues – and so-called 'healthy' foods continue to emerge into the marketplace at an alarming rate. More and more sugar-laden breakfast cereals, for example, have recently found their way to our supermarket shelves. It's a rarity to find a full-fat, sugar free yoghurt product – virtually all are low-fat with added sugars. Snacks are invariably carb-based and low-fat.

But the fact is that our modern understanding of nutrition is based on a science that is *not* yet complete. More and more information is emerging about the chemical make-up of food and how that affects our bodies. Not only is the science incomplete, it is young – it is still evolving!

The 1930s was a decade of real nutritional discovery. You may be surprised to learn that vitamins, minerals, and the essentiality of fats were all unknown before then. The 'omega' group of fatty acids was not even named until the mid-1960s.

As research reveals and confirms new knowledge, much of our previous understanding is now being overturned. Much of our thinking about what constitutes a 'healthy' diet - even though it is only a few decades old – is already obsolete!

What was knowledge only a few years ago is already relegated to food mythology. Let's remind ourselves that the Harvard School of Public Health already considers '*it's time to end the low-fat myth*'! Low-fat already a myth? For many of us, this has been a perceived wisdom for most of our adult lives. After a few short decades, the errors of that supposed wisdom have come to light, though the vast majority have yet to catch up with **'the 6 diet'**!

So let's take a look at the very latest thinking, knowledge and understanding about brought to you for the first time by **'the 6 diet'**.

About nutrients

Let's look at a few definitions - a nutrient is:

- a substance that provides nourishment essential for growth and the maintenance of life

- a chemical that an organism needs to live and grow or a substance used in an organism's metabolism which must be taken in from its environment
- a chemical compound that makes up the food organisms need to survive

OK – so nutrients are necessary for our survival, growth and maintenance. Now, I want you to honestly answer these questions...

When you eat something, is your primary motivation about survival, growth and maintenance, or is to satisfy hunger, taste or emotional indulgence? When preparing your meal do you think about eating what you fancy, or what your body needs? Do you eat what is convenient or what is useful?

The truth is probably a little bit of all those things. Whilst we certainly are drawn towards great tasting food – whatever that means to each of us – we also undoubtedly try to do what is good for us. By the very fact that you are reading this, you are interested in eating as healthily as you can. In my clinical work I have seen many people who really try to adopt healthy eating habits, but who fail to benefit because the information they are working from is fundamentally flawed. I used to be just like that too!

Most 'diets' fail to address the issue of what different foods do for us. Instead they focus on achieving a result – such as weight loss – without any regard for what that means to an individual in terms of their overall health. Worse are those sectors of the diet industry whose real purpose is to promote their own food products which are nutritionally lacking. Sadly, many consumers are led to buy really dreadful products and so called ready-meals believing they are doing themselves some good.

'the 6 diet' suggests that there is nothing better for you than fresh, well-cooked produce. Forget anything tampered with in a laboratory; forget additives, preservatives, and anything else artificial. These things are simply not food – they have no place in a healthy body!

The key to a great body, great figure, vibrant health and vitality, is good nutrition. It provides the building blocks of everything we are. Since sailors discovered that citrus could keep scurvy at bay we have been aware of the intimate relationship between food and health. In this section we are going to take a journey of discovery of our own. We will identify basic nutritional needs, and how to satisfy them.

Macro and micro nutrients

The only things we need to concentrate on are real nutrients. Some nutrients are needed in relatively large quantities – these are called 'macronutrients'. Some are needed in respectively smaller quantities – these are called 'micronutrients'.

Macro nutrients

By now these will be familiar to you. The macro nutrients are:

- Proteins
- Fats
- Carbohydrates
- Water

We have already looked at some aspects of these, so let's add to our knowledge about them.

Proteins

Some basics about proteins

Protein is found throughout our bodies. It is a component of our muscles, bones, skin, hair, and virtually every other body part, tissue or cell. It makes up some special substances called 'enzymes' that power the chemical reactions needed in the body. For example, our pancreases produce enzymes to help to break down and digest the foods that we eat: the process of breaking those chemical bonds between sugar molecules in carbohydrates is done by enzymes. The haemoglobin that carries oxygen in our blood also contains protein. In fact our DNA itself is protein!

At least 10,000 different proteins make us what we are and keep us that way: we need dietary protein to provide the materials necessary to develop, grow, repair and maintain all the bodily tissues and substances made up of protein.

In the same way that complex carbohydrates are made up of chains of sugar molecules, protein is also made up of chains of basic building blocks: these are called amino acids. Sources differ about exact numbers, but fundamentally there are about twenty known amino acids that provide the raw material for all proteins. Some amino acids can be manufactured from elements within our own bodies, but fourteen of them cannot. These fourteen, which are therefore called 'essential amino acids', must be delivered to our bodies through the food that we eat. Whenever we see the word 'essential' in relation to nutrients, they must be provided through food because our bodies cannot make them for us.

Because the body doesn't store amino acids, as it does fats or carbohydrates, it needs a daily supply of amino acids to make new protein.

All protein foods are not equal: equal that is in terms of their respective values to our bodies. Some of the protein we eat contains all the amino acids needed to build new proteins. This kind is called 'complete' protein. Animal sources of protein, such as meat, fish, poultry, eggs etc. tend to be complete. Other protein sources lack one or more of the essential amino acids. Called 'incomplete' proteins, these usually come from fruits, vegetables, grains, and nuts.

Vegetarians need to be very aware of this. To get all the amino acids needed to make new protein and keep our bodies in good shape and functioning well can be tricky. If you don't eat meat, fish, poultry, eggs, or dairy products you have to learn how to combine different vegetarian protein foods each day to ensure the full range of amino acids are consumed. Brown rice and beans, for example, is one way that we can combine foods to ensure we get our full complement.

While the nutritional value of the proteins themselves delivered from animal or vegetable sources probably have the same effects on our health, the other nutrient components of these different types may make a difference however. For example, animal-based protein foods also tend to provide us with a much higher dose of saturated fats. Vegetable sources of protein, such as beans, nuts, and whole grains, are excellent choices, and they offer healthy fibre, vitamins, and minerals. Nuts are also a great source of healthy fats. We'll talk more about fats shortly.

A lack of protein can be a serious matter. Growth failure, loss of muscle mass, decreased immunity, weakening of the heart and weakening of the respiratory system, even death, can result from insufficient protein.

The amount of protein that we need depends on our size. The Harvard School of Public Health advises that adults need a minimum of 0.8 grams of protein for every kilogram (or about 20lbs) of body weight every day just to keep us from breaking down our own bodily tissues. This is a rough average though, and differs in children, pregnancy etc., so these figures shouldn't be taken as right for everyone: remember, there is no good 'one-size-fits-all' advice where diet is concerned!

So, to summarise what we already know about proteins:

- They are made up of chains of amino acids
- Some amino acids are 'essential' – so called because our bodies cannot manufacture them and we have to obtain them from our diets
- Some amino acids are non-essential – which means that our bodies can make them from other

nutrients within our diets

- 🔊 Some proteins are 'complete' – so called because they contain all the different amino acids that our bodies need
- 🔊 Some are 'incomplete' – because they lack one or more of the amino acids that our bodies need
- 🔊 They are large molecules, and take a relatively high amount of digestive time and effort
- 🔊 They can help to even out the rate at which our bodies digest carbohydrates, and therefore help to balance our blood sugar
- 🔊 They are needed for development, growth, repair and maintenance of all of our bodily tissues
- 🔊 They are needed for our bodies to make vital substances, such as hormones, enzymes etc.
- 🔊 We need to eat proteins every day because our bodies cannot store amino acids for future use

Hopefully, the information above is all we need to give us some motivation to eat protein-rich foods. Every day!

So where do we find our protein?

There are two basic sources of proteins. Some are from animal-based foods, and some are plant-based.

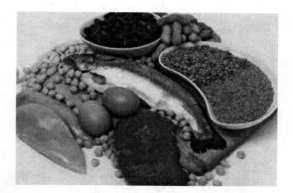

🔊 **Fish and Seafood**

Most seafood is very low in fat, which makes it a particularly good source of protein. Some fish, like salmon, has a lot of fat, but it is the good type. Being an animal-based source, it contains all the essential amino acids, and is therefore a complete protein source.

Meat

All meats are sources of complete protein. Red meats are renowned for their high levels of high-calorie saturated fats, so it isn't wise to make this your only or main source of proteins.

Poultry

This is a great provider of protein because it is very lean. The dark meat is a little higher in fat than white meat. Beware though: the skin on poultry is loaded with saturated fat.

Dairy products, including milk, cheese, yoghurt, cream etc.

These products are sources of complete protein. However, nutritionally the picture is very mixed: they contain some good nutrients in terms of minerals and vitamins, but often have high levels of saturated fats too. Cows' milk products tend to be the most commonly used in many parts of the world, but are thought to promote inflammation, being linked with some inflammatory diseases and conditions. However, goat and sheep milk products are generally less fatty, and generally considered to be less damaging than cows' milk products.

Eggs

These are high in protein but very low in calories. One egg provides about 7g of complete protein, and its amino acid profile is considered to be optimum. What a great food! (One of the obsolete pieces of information that we can now discard is that eggs are a problem for cholesterol: simply not true!)

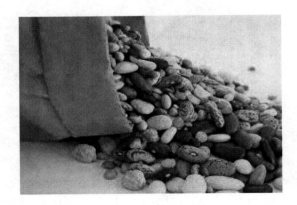

- **Mycoproteins**

  Mycoproteins are found in meat-substitute products, and are generally vegan sources of protein (i.e. they are totally plant-based and contain no animal-based nutrients at all).

- **Soya**

  Soya protein is one of the few plant proteins that contains all of the essential amino acids, and is therefore a complete protein food. It is generally low in fat.

- **Nuts**

  These do not contain all the essential amino acids, and therefore need to be combined with other foods. They are, however, a great source of several vitamins and important minerals.

- **Pulses / legumes, including beans, chickpeas, lentils etc.**

  These contain a higher proportion of protein than most other plant foods and they are low in fat. However they are deficient in one of the essential amino acids, Methionine, so do not provide complete protein.

- **Grains/cereals**

  The proteins found in grains and cereals tend to be deficient in the essential amino acid Lycine. And we should remember that grains and cereals are increasingly linked with inflammation, which makes them one of the least healthy choices.

- **Seeds**

  These are incomplete proteins, but are a good source of a range of useful vitamins and minerals.

For meat-eaters, it isn't a problem to obtain the complete complement of amino acids in your diet. Vegetarians have to ensure a range of protein-based foods are consumed to ensure a full complement of amino acids.

Fats

Some basic facts about fats

More correctly we might call fats either 'lipids' or 'fatty acids'.

Like proteins, fats are also vital to our health. They have received so much bad press over so many years that it's really difficult to think of them as nutrients. Many of us have been conditioned by the diet and weight-loss industry to think that 'low-fat' or even 'fat-free' is beneficial and that dietary fat is harmful. Indeed, in my clinical experience I have worked with patients who really struggle at first to accept the concept that fat is a good thing.

Sarah, a patient who successfully completed **'the 6 diet'** and achieved great body changing results explains how her journey didn't begin the way she expected:

> *"I was completely surprised to not be buying or eating low-fat foods, because this is what I've been doing for years, following mainstream advice. At first it felt completely alien, and took me about 2 weeks to really get my head around it. My views of food have completely changed following my experience of **'the 6 diet'** and I have learned where I was going wrong. I feel so much healthier and energetic, and I lost several inches of body fat. I now understand why having the right information is crucial to getting fantastic results".*

The Harvard School of Public Health agree, insisting *'It's time to end the low-fat myth'*. Hurrah!

Let's take a closer look at what they have to say about dietary fats (published on their website 2012:

> *"'Low-fa',' 'reduced fat', or 'fat-free' processed foods are not necessarily 'healthy', nor is it automatically healthier to follow a low-fat diet. One problem with a generic lower-fat diet is that it prompts most people to stop eating fats that are good for the heart along with those that are bad for it. And low-fat diets are often higher in refined carbohydrates and starches from foods like white rice, white bread, potatoes, and sugary drinks. Similarly, when food manufacturers take out fat, they often replace it with carbohydrates from sugar, refined grains, or starch. Our bodies digest these refined carbohydrates and starches very quickly, causing blood sugar and insulin levels to spike and then dip, which in turn leads to hunger, overeating, and weight gain. Over time, eating lots of 'fast carbs' can raise the risk of heart disease and diabetes as much as—or more than—eating too much saturated fat."*

Now that really sounds like **'the 6 diet'** to me!

I've already mentioned that low-fat food products equal high-refined-carb-products, and the inherent problems that causes for our blood sugar balance. But Harvard raises another great point. If you severely limit your fat intake, you deprive your own body of some vital nutrients too. Many of the healthy tissues in our bodies have a fat component: in part we are made of fat. In fact some really important parts of our bodies are made of fat. Our brains and nervous systems (spinal column and nerve sheaths etc.), both have significant fat components. So when you take fats out of your diet, you deprive your body of some of the vital building blocks to grow, repair and maintain these vital bodily structures!

Hopefully 'low-fat' and 'fat-free' are sounding much less attractive now?!

Good and bad fats

Of course, there are indeed 'good' fats and 'bad' fats. The fats we should think of as good are technically the 'monounsaturated' and 'polyunsaturated' fats. These are thought to actually lower our risk of developing disease.

For decades we have been led to believe that saturated fats are unhealthy. However, recent thinking casts doubt on that assumption. Certainly it is sensible to limit saturated fats – they are high in calories, and in excess can certainly contribute to overweight and obesity. BUT it has been shown that they don't necessarily contribute to disease conditions as previously thought – indeed one of the fats now been promoted as a healthy option for cooking is coconut oil – rich in saturated fat!

Truly 'bad' fats are technically the 'trans fats'. These certainly increase our disease risk. It's worth taking a closer look at trans fats – sometimes called hydrogenated fats. They are often found in foods that masquerade as 'healthy' food products, such as vegetable oil-based spreads etc. These fats are laboratory-made products, not found in *any* natural food. They are often made so that you can spread a vegetable fat. But think for a moment – VEGETABLE FATS ARE LIQUID AT ROOM TEMPERATURE. They all tend to be pourable: olive oil, sunflower oil, sesame oil, walnut oil, etc.

Nature didn't make them solid so scientists did!

Liquid oils are made solid and spreadable by adding extra hydrogen into the chemical structure of the fat molecules: this gives them their name 'hydrogen-ated'. At the end of this they are no longer the same chemical product as the original fat, and are not recognisable to our bodies.

They are particularly dangerous to our health because we have no means to digest or process them.

TRANS FATS ARE NOT FOOD! They have no place in our bodies!

A word about cholesterol

Cholesterol is also a fat, and enjoys a poor reputation that it doesn't necessarily deserve. In the past we have been advised to severely reduce or limit the amount of cholesterol we take in our diets. However, for most people, unless there is a specific medical problem, dietary cholesterol isn't the villain it's been portrayed to be. Cholesterol in the bloodstream is what's most important, but that is made by our own livers, it isn't generally the cholesterol that we eat. The biggest influence on blood cholesterol level is the mix of fats and carbohydrates in our diet - not the amount of cholesterol we eat from food. So eggs, which have previously suffered from the poor reputation that was wrongly given to foods containing cholesterol can now enjoy a new popularity!

Could it be that we've been misled about the dangers of high cholesterol? Well let's take a look at what cholesterol is, and what we now know it does for us. Essentially cholesterol is one of our bodies' repair mechanisms, and it responds to inflammatory damage in our blood vessels. When the body detects such damage, it sends cholesterol to the damaged site. If left to its own devices cholesterol attaches itself over the damaged area in the vessel wall, and gradually becomes absorbed to create a newly smooth section. Of course, if there is too much inflammation, causing too much damage then we see high levels of cholesterol appearing in our blood stream – it's there to help. I could expand on the mechanisms involved with cholesterol, and the potential dangers of lowering its levels without tackling the underlying problems of inflammation, but that's a whole other book!

What we need to understand here is that the common link between inflammation and a whole variety of diseases is how people who develop type 2 diabetes go on to develop high cholesterol, or vice versa. It's not so much that one disease causes the other, but rather that they share a common cause – inflammation! And it's the inflammation that needs to be tackled in order to help both conditions.

Essential fatty acids

As with amino acids, some fatty acids are essential – remember that means they must be consumed as part of our diet because our bodies cannot manufacture them for us. These include the omega fats identified and named only a few short decades ago: think especially here of omegas 3 and 6. It's really important to understand a little about these fats, because they are intrinsically linked with inflammation: especially crucial given the emerging understanding of diabetes as an inflammatory disease!

Let's take a moment to understand inflammation. Inflammation isn't always a bad thing – in fact it can be a life-saver. We all need an inflammatory response mechanism. Let's say we cut ourselves on a dirty object. What is it that prevents or fights infection that may enter directly through an open wound? The answer is the inflammatory response – raising the temperature at the site of the wound, and flooding the area with specialist cells geared up to combat infectious germs.

The problem with inflammation comes when our inflammatory response is initiated unnecessarily, or doesn't switch off. The inflammatory response turns its unwelcome attention onto our own bodily tissues, creating any of a range of disease conditions, including serious autoimmune illnesses: rheumatism, rheumatoid arthritis, lupus to name a few.

Omega-6 fatty acids are a part of the inflammatory mechanism in the body – being a key nutrient to fuel our bodies' inflammatory response. Omega-3, on the other hand, is a key nutrient to combat inflammation – it is anti-inflammatory in nature. In antiquity the human diet delivered a ratio of approximately 1:1 Omega-6 to Omega-3. That is no longer the case. Our modern processed diets deliver much higher rations of Omega-6 to Omega-3 and as such contribute to excess inflammatory factors in the human body, and contributing to many diseases and conditions associated with inflammation – including diabetes according to the latest thinking! We should, therefore, be very careful to limit the amount of Omega-6 fatty acids that we consume. Avoiding Omega-6 rich fats and oils in favour of those rich in Omega-3, and ensuring a smaller ratio of these essential nutrients is crucial.

So where fats are concerned, the key to a healthy diet is to choose dietary fats carefully. Our bodies can cope well with moderate amounts of saturated fats, found in butter and some plant-based fats such as coconut and brazil nuts. Oils rich in Omega-3 fatty acids are especially important: think olive oil, one of the key nutritional components of the beneficial Mediterranean diet. On the other hand, Omega-6 fatty acids should be kept to a minimum to prevent inappropriate inflammation: think sunflower oil, rapeseed/canola oils. Trans/hydrogenated fats should be completely avoided – the dangers of these compounds are now well known and researched! And finally, unless you have a specific medical need, you don't have to pay too much attention to the amount of cholesterol present in your food. It's time to think about many fats as friends instead of always treating them as dietary foes!

Again, let's first of all summarise what we already know about fats:

- There are good fats and bad fats
- The really good fats are monounsaturated and polyunsaturated – though we need to take care with over-consumption of those rich in Omega-6
- Saturated fats have enjoyed bad press and are generally considered to be bad fats – but remember our bodies can cope with small amounts: they improve satiety, staving off hunger, but their high-calorific nature might help us to gain weight if not kept to moderate levels
- The very worst fats are trans fats or hydrogenated fats, and should be completely avoided
- Some fats are essential – i.e. we have to obtain them from our diets
- A large proportion of our bodily tissues are made of fat, making them a crucial part of our diets
- Like proteins, fats can slow down the rate of carbohydrate metabolism, making us feel fuller for longer

Let's not be fearful of fats any longer. All we need to know is where to get our good fats, and how to avoid the bad ones, which fats are essential, and which are not, and which fats can actually heal us and improve our health.

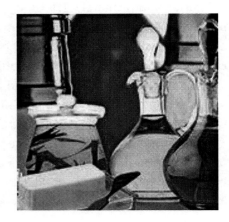

Monounsaturated Fats

Many vegetable oils are rich in monounsaturated fats. Those with the highest monounsaturated fatty acid content include olive, avocado, almond, peanut, corn, sesame, rice bran, soybean and cod liver oils. Hazelnuts, macadamia nuts, pecans, almonds, pistachios and cashews are rich food sources of monounsaturated fats. Butters made from these nuts are therefore also great sources.

Only two fruits - avocados and olives - are rich sources of monounsaturated fats.

Peanuts are the legume that is richest in monounsaturated fats. Peanut butter is also an excellent food source of this fat.

Sesame seeds, as well as sesame seed butter or paste (tahini), is high in monounsaturated fatty acids. Sunflower seeds (and sunflower seed butter), pumpkin and flaxseeds provide some monounsaturated fat.

Polyunsaturated Fats

All cooking and salad oils contain a mixture of the various fatty acids -- monounsaturated, polyunsaturated and saturated, so don't be confused if some foods appear on more than one list!

The oils that are richest in polyunsaturated fatty acids include sesame, safflower, soybean, corn and sunflower-seed oils.

Legumes, such as peanuts and peanut butter, contain a blend of unsaturated fatty acids but are a good food source of polyunsaturated fatty acids. Soybeans are rich in polyunsaturated fatty acids as well. Over half of the fat in soybeans is polyunsaturated.

Pumpkin seeds, sesame seeds and sesame seed butter are all food sources of polyunsaturated fats. However, aside from flax seeds, sunflower seeds contain the most polyunsaturated fatty acids. Approximately 75 percent of the fat in these seeds is polyunsaturated.

Omega-3 Fats

Omega-3 fats are healthy polyunsaturated types. The three most nutritionally important Omega-3 fatty acids are alpha-linolenic acid, eicosapentaenoic acid (EPA) and docosahexaenoic acid (DHA).

There are some animal-based sources and some plant-based sources.

DHA and EPA are found in fatty, cold water fish including salmon, mackerel, halibut, sardines, tuna and herring and are generally considered to be the most beneficial to our bodies. DHA is concentrated in the brain and in the retinas of the eyes, and is crucial for proper brain and nerve development. EPA doesn't become part of the brain's structure, but does reduce inflammatory processes in the brain and has a unique role of maintaining a healthy mood, as well as playing a role in the prevention of cardiovascular diseases.

ALA is the plant-based form of Omega-3 and is found in some vegetables like kale and spinach, flax and pumpkin seeds and walnuts. It is important for heart health. The body converts ALA into EPA and DHA, but not terribly efficiently. Therefore, some people consider that vegetarians are missing out on important EPA and DHA fats. However, these are found in such high levels in fish due to the diets of the fish: algae! Certain types of algae contain DHA. Vegetarians who are unwilling to take fish oils into their diet may benefit from ALA-rich foods, such as flaxseed oils, combined with an algae food source or supplement to promote the conversion of ALA into EPA and DHA.

So here are some great reasons to be eating Omega-3 fats including:
- o To reduce inflammation throughout your body
- o To keep your blood from clotting excessively
- o To maintain your cell membranes
- o To lower the amount of fats, such as cholesterol and triglycerides, in your bloodstream
- o To prevent hardening of your arteries
- o To enable your arteries to relax and dilate
- o To reduce your risk of becoming obese
- o To improve your insulin response and help to balance your blood sugar
- o To help you prevent cancer cell growth

Omega-6 Fats

Omega-6 fatty acids are also polyunsaturated fats. They are also essential, and otherwise called linoleic acid.

They are found in seeds and nuts, and the oils extracted from them, such as sunflower, maize / corn, safflower. They are also found in eggs and meat and dairy products. Where there are only a few sources of Omega-3 in our typical diets, sources of Omega-6 fatty acids are numerous. Many refined vegetable oils, used in most snack foods, are rich in Omega-6.

Our bodies use Omega-6 fatty acids to make hormones. In general, hormones from Omega-6 fatty acids tend to increase inflammation. As we have already discussed, we all need an inflammatory response as part of our immune system. The hormones made from Omega-3 fatty acids decrease inflammation. Both families of hormones must be in balance to maintain our optimum health.

Many nutrition experts believe that before we relied so heavily on processed foods, we would have consumed Omega-3 and Omega-6 fatty acids in roughly equal amounts. But to our great detriment, we now get far too much of the Omega-6s and not enough of the Omega-3s. This dietary imbalance may explain the increase of such diseases as asthma, coronary heart disease, many forms of cancer, autoimmunity and neurodegenerative diseases, all of which are believed to stem from inflammation in the body. There is some evidence that an imbalance between Omega-3 and Omega-6 fatty acids may also contribute to obesity, depression, dyslexia, hyperactivity and even a tendency toward violence.

Ensuring we consume these fats in a healthy proportion is therefore crucial. Because we can readily get Omega-6 in our diets we rarely need to think about supplementing it. However, the opposite may well be true of Omega-3. Care should be taken to ensure you don't eat foods that are too high in Omega-6: oils like sunflower and rapeseed are thought to have the balance wrong for example!

Saturated Fats

Now we are getting into the realms of those fats that we are often told we need to severely limit or avoid. They have previously been associated with a range of diseases – such as cardiovascular diseases and strokes, cancers etc., partly because saturated fats raise total and bad (LDL) cholesterol levels. However, recent research indicates that saturated fat is not as bad as previously thought. Indeed, coconut oil is currently being promoted as a healthy option for cooking!

What appears to be more important than avoiding saturated fat, is incorporating more Omega-3 fats into our diets! Again this is a surprising 'new' finding in the nutrition world.

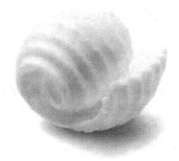

The main sources of saturated fat are from animal products: red meat and whole-milk dairy products, including cheese, sour cream, ice cream and butter. There are also plant-based sources of saturated fat, principally coconut oil and coconut milk, palm kernel oil, cocoa butter, and palm oil. Several of these are typically found in prepared food products. Whilst cocoa butter is in chocolate, coconut oil and palm oils are found in many bakery products.

'the 6 diet' advice about saturated fats is that since we don't actually need them there is no real reason to consume them. But we shouldn't be afraid of them in moderate amounts. Your body will, after all, cope quite well with a small amount.

🙢 Trans Fats or Hydrogenated Fats

Avoid, avoid, avoid. At all costs!

These extremely harmful fats have been used recklessly in the food industry for many years. Since 2006 it has been a legal requirement in some countries to clearly show them on food labels. Since that time the food industry has also seen fit to find alternatives within food products. That tells us something powerful! When they finally had to be open about the use of trans fats, the food industry stopped using them so much: the dangers of using them must indeed be high!

Trans fats are made by a chemical process called partial hydrogenation. Liquid vegetable oils – many of which, in their natural state, are ironically amongst the healthiest types of fats - are packed with hydrogen atoms and converted into a solid fat. The food industry likes to work with trans fats because of their high melting point, creamy, smooth texture and reusability in deep-fat frying. These fats also extend the shelf life of food.

So why are they considered to be so unhealthy?

Remember the liver processes fats. Because it can never break down trans fats it keeps processing, and processing and processing, and eventually this activity gives rise to the production of bad (LDL) cholesterol, whilst stripping our levels of good (HDL) cholesterol, the kind that actually helps unclog our arteries. Trans fats also increase triglyceride levels in the blood, adding to our risk of cardiovascular disease.

Carbohydrates

We have already covered carbohydrates in great depth in previous sections. Let's recap what we already know:

- 🙢 There are two basic categories of carbohydrate: simple / refined and complex.
- 🙢 The most simple carbohydrates are sugars
- 🙢 Carbohydrates are the main fuel source for our bodies
- 🙢 Digestion works to turn all carbohydrates into glucose, which is what our bodies need for energy

- The more simple the carbohydrate, the faster the body can convert it to glucose
- Complex carbohydrates take between 1 and 3 hours to be converted into sugars
- Some glucose is vital for our brain function: without it we will die
- Most of the glucose we use is as a result of our bodies digesting carbohydrates, not from eating glucose itself
- Too many sugars and refined carbohydrates are linked with insulin resistance, a precursor to type 2 diabetes
- Too many sugars and refined carbohydrates are linked with leptin resistance, which causes us to store more visceral fat, and eventually increases our risk of developing type 2 diabetes

The best carbohydrates are as natural and unprocessed as possible. You should select whole grains (in moderation according to your activity levels and energy needs), vegetables, fruits and beans. Not only do they provide us with slow-release complex carbohydrates, but they promote good health by delivering vitamins, minerals, fibre and a host of important plant-based nutrients. You should avoid the rapidly digested carbohydrates from refined grains - such as white bread, white rice, etc. - as well as sugary or sweetened foods - cakes, pastries, biscuits, sweets, sugary drinks and beverages - and other highly processed foods.

Such refined carbohydrate foods contribute to weight gain, interfere with weight loss, and promote type 2 diabetes, heart disease etc.

It is probably quite shocking to hear that, after years of being programmed to believe that low-fat foods are a healthy choice, recent research warns us that diets high in refined carbohydrates are more dangerous and damaging to our health than diets high in saturated fats. That's a real turn-around in nutritional thinking, but hopefully, having read Chapters 1 and 2 of this book you'll be much more familiar with this concept now!

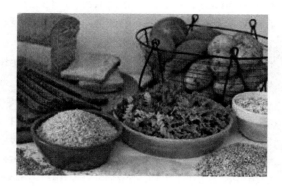

Carbohydrates that are typically NOT very useful in our diets include:
- Bread

- Potatoes
- Pasta
- White rice
- Tortillas / wraps made with white flour
- Breadsticks
- Biscuits, cookies, cakes, pastries
- Pizza dough

More useful carbohydrates include:

- Vegetables – especially the green, leafy varieties
- Beans
- Legumes / pulses such as chickpeas, lentils etc.
- Nuts
- Seeds
- Whole grain cereals, such as oats, oatmeal, barley, millet, spelt and rye
- Brown or wild rice

So much of a typical western diet is carbohydrate-based, and we really need to be cautious about the over-consumption of carbohydrate foods. We don't need nearly as many cereal-based or grain-based foods as we once imagined, or indeed have come to use by habit. Previous dietetic advice has suggested that 40-60% of a meal should be made up of carbohydrate – absolutely not! Not for general health for most people living a modern lifestyle and definitely not for anyone who is at risk or has already developed diabetes! As I write, a review of this advice, by NHS and other healthcare professionals, is way overdue – until it happens vulnerable patients will continue to receive improper advice.

Toast for breakfast, a sandwich for lunch, pasta / rice / potatoes with our evening meal: too much, far too much! Rather we should significantly reduce cereals and grains in favour of wholesome fresh vegetables, pulses / legumes, nuts, seeds etc. In this way we take advantage of the much wider range of proteins, minerals, vitamins and other nutrients that **'the 6 diet'** reminds us that we should consume.

Water

Maybe it's a surprise to consider water as a vital nutrient. But that's exactly what it is! Without it we would die, and much more quickly than by depriving ourselves of other nutrients.

We have already talked a little about the way in which our bodies use water, so let's remind ourselves of what we already know:

- 🕮 Water is required within each of our bodily cells
- 🕮 It is transported across our cell membranes
- 🕮 Water inside our cells is called hydration
- 🕮 Water that accumulates on the outside of cells is called water retention

Water makes up about 50 to 70 per cent of an adult's total body weight. Without regular top-ups we would fail to survive for more than just a few days.

It is an essential requirement for our bodies' growth and maintenance, and is involved in a number of bodily processes. For example, it helps us get rid of waste from our bodies; it regulates our temperature, and it provides the means for lots of biochemical processes to occur. Quite simply, every cell in our bodies needs water to function properly.

We regularly lose water through urine and sweat, and therefore it must be replaced through our diet. If we don't take in enough we risk dehydration. Maybe surprisingly, just a 1% decrease in hydration can lead to an 8%-10% decrease in bodily performance. Dehydration is being linked, through research, with serious illnesses from back and joint pains, to some cancers. When we are dehydrated our concentration levels, reaction times and even strength can decrease. But it's not just our performance that is affected. We may also experience symptoms such as headaches, tiredness and loss of mental ability. Also our appearance may begin to suffer – we need water to maintain a healthy complexion and skin.

Water is also crucial for weight management. We need water to help our bodies rid themselves of toxins, as it is the main carrier that helps us flush them out. Much of our blood stream is made of water. Our blood delivers all the nutrients and oxygen to our cells but it also takes all the toxins and waste away. If we are dehydrated then our kidneys don't function properly, potentially leading to constipation and kidney stones and resulting in an excess work load being placed on our livers. As a result, we end up re-absorbing toxins into our fat cells and also slowing down the rate we can burn off our body fat. To help you lose weight, drink more water.

Consuming too little water also leads to fluid retention! If we are restricting our water supply then our bodies try to keep hold of any fluid we already have. It may sound counterintuitive, but if you know that you retain water, drink more of it!

We obtain our fluid from three main sources:

- Drinks, either plain water or as part of other beverages including tea, coffee and squash
- Solid foods, especially fruit and vegetables (even foods such as bread and cheese provide small amounts of fluid)
- As a by-product of chemical reactions within our bodies

Most healthy adults need between one and a half to three litres of water each day, so we should aim to drink six to eight medium glasses of water daily. Some beverages can count towards our fluid intake, but others, especially those containing sugars or caffeine, can actually cause the opposite effect because they promote water retention rather than proper hydration. Of course, in hot weather, or when we are especially physically active, and may lose more water through sweating, we need to consume more.

Our bodies can confuse dehydration for hunger. If you know you are eating plenty of food, yet still feel hungry, it may be that you are really thirsty: in the first instance then, drink more water.

While it is true that our bodies can obtain water from beverages and foods, **'the 6 diet'** tells us that pure, clean water is what we really need, and that there really is no substitute for that!

Micro nutrients

The micronutrients are those that our bodies typically need in small doses! Essentially, these are the vitamins and minerals and antioxidants that we need to promote and maintain good health.

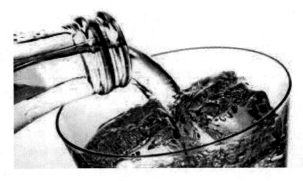

Until the 1930s these were actually undiscovered. However, even though the vitamins and minerals themselves hadn't been identified, our ancestors had realised centuries previously that deficiencies in these nutrients caused illness, and that ensuring we consumed them prevented and even cured those specifically related illnesses. For example, we typically associate a deficiency of Vitamin C with scurvy; a deficiency of Vitamin D with rickets; a deficiency of iron with anaemia etc.

Therefore, consuming a diet that delivers a full complement of micronutrients in appropriate amounts and ratios is essential for our health and well-being.

Let's familiarise ourselves with what they are, what they do, and where we can find them!

Vitamins

Fundamentally, there are two categories of vitamins. There are some fat-soluble vitamins, and some water-soluble vitamins. The fat soluble vitamins are best taken in a fatty medium, such as with a drink of milk, to promote their absorption into our bodies. We have a capacity to store some excess fat-soluble vitamins in our own fatty tissues – which of course is one of the reasons why we all need a certain amount of body fat. This does mean, however, that we can effectively 'overdose' on fat-soluble vitamins, leading to a build-up of toxic proportions within our bodies. Water soluble vitamins, on the other hand, are better taken with a drink of water. We have no ability to store them, and any excess is excreted from our bodies in our faeces or urine.

The fat-soluble vitamins are A, D, E and K. The water soluble vitamins are the B's and C. We'll take a look at these in turn:

Vitamin A

Why do you need it?	Where do you find it?
🔹 Skin repair: includes mucous membranes 🔹 Bones and teeth 🔹 Enhances immunity 🔹 Digestive health (heals ulcers) 🔹 Protects against heart disease / strokes, and lowers cholesterol 🔹 Slows the ageing process	🔹 Animal livers 🔹 Fish livers – e.g. cod liver oil 🔹 Carotenes from red / yellow / green vegetables (body makes Vitamin A from beta carotenes) ** You can take too much vitamin A and it can accumulate in the body because it is stored in the liver and fatty tissues. Zinc helps prevent build up.

Vitamin D

Why do you need it?	Where do you find it?
🔆 Muscle strength 🔆 Bones and teeth – including protection against osteoporosis and osteoarthritis 🔆 Enhances immunity 🔆 Regulates heartbeat 🔆 Protects against breast cancer, colon cancer 🔆 Normal blood clotting 🔆 Thyroid function 🔆 Stabilises nervous system	🔆 Animal livers 🔆 Fish livers and oily fish – e.g. cod liver oil 🔆 Sweet potatoes 🔆 Eggs 🔆 Dairy products ** Calcium is required alongside vitamin D.

Vitamin E

Why do you need it?	Where do you find it?
🔆 Circulation: prevents too much blood clotting, dilates blood vessels, lowers cholesterol deposits, prevents varicose veins 🔆 Protects against heart disease, lowers blood pressure (diuretic action) 🔆 Slows ageing process 🔆 Aids immune system 🔆 Regulates menstruation 🔆 Helps other nutrients' actions	🔆 Whole grains 🔆 Leafy vegetables 🔆 Vegetable oils 🔆 Fish 🔆 Eggs 🔆 Nuts and seeds ** Take with selenium

Vitamin K

Why do you need it?	Where do you find it?
Blood clotting	Kelp
Normal liver function	Alfalfa
	Green vegetables
	Fish liver oils
	Dairy products
	Eggs
	Molasses
	Intestinal bacteria

Vitamin B

Here it is worth pointing out that there are several different B vitamins within the family. Each has its own associated illnesses and purposes. However, they do have some commonality, and for our purpose of giving a brief overview these have been combined in our table below:

Why do you need it?	Where do you find it?
Metabolism: energy from food	Brown rice, whole grains,
Support vital functions: heart, brain, nervous system, muscle functions, digestive system	Yeast, molasses
Growth and development	Nuts and seeds
Production of blood cells and bone marrow	Pulses/legumes
Production of hormones	Meat and fish
Fluid balance	Eggs
Skin and hair	Dairy and soya milk products
	Dried fruits, dates
	Green vegetables: especially kale, broccoli and spinach
	Seaweeds
	Intestinal bacteria (B8) – *one of the things that makes them 'good bacteria'*

Vitamin C

Why do you need it?	Where do you find it?
☙ Blood vessels	☙ Fresh fruit: guava, kiwi, currants
☙ Muscles	☙ Fruit juices
☙ Bones, teeth, gums	☙ Peppers
☙ Enhances immunity, anti-bacterial, anti-viral	☙ Brussels sprouts
☙ Promotes wound healing, skin	** Best taken with magnesium or calcium rather than as ascorbic acid

As you will no doubt appreciate from studying the tables above, consuming your full range of vitamins really means having a varied and interesting diet, rich in great tasting fresh produce!

Minerals

We need a wide range of minerals in our diet in order to protect and promote our good health. Some we need in terms of milligrams, other in the much smaller micrograms. These are present in our bodies in very tiny amounts: it is estimated that about 60 different minerals make up about 4% of our normal body weight. Some are considered essential.

Let's take a closer look at fifteen of the most common and necessary minerals:

Calcium

Why do you need it?	Signs of possible deficiency	Where do you find it?
☙ Healthy bones & teeth	☙ Muscle aches and pains	☙ Whitebait
☙ Helps control blood cholesterol levels	☙ Cramps	☙ Bones in canned fish
☙ Nerve function	☙ Poor bone density	☙ Sesame seeds
☙ Muscle function	☙ Early onset of cataracts	☙ Dairy products
☙ Digestive function		☙ Soya beans
☙ Regulates heart muscle		☙ Nuts
☙ Regulates sleep		☙ Broccoli
☙ Helps with absorption of Vitamin B12		☙ Green leafy vegetables
		☙ Seaweeds
		☙ Pulses / legumes

		<ul><li>Whole grains</li><li>Oranges</li></ul>

The most absorbable form of calcium is as citrate. Its absorption is aided by magnesium, vitamin D and lactose. Its absorption is hindered by phytates (from wheat), caffeine, oxalic acid (found in rhubarb and spinach), saturated fats, salt and sugar.

Chloride

Why do you need it?	Signs of possible deficiency	Where do you find it?
<ul><li>Required for the formation of acids in the stomach</li><li>Regulating fluid in all blood vessels</li><li>Regulating fluid in all cells</li></ul>	<ul><li>Low blood pressure</li><li>** Deficiencies are very rare.</li></ul>	<ul><li>Table salt</li><li>Other foods containing sodium chloride</li></ul>

Chromium

Why do you need it?	Signs of possible deficiency	Where do you find it?
<ul><li>Stabilise blood sugar levels</li><li>Prevent diabetes, by using insulin efficiently</li><li>Aids the break-down of fats in the body</li><li>Regulates cholesterol</li></ul>	<ul><li>Cravings for sugar or sweet foods</li></ul>	<ul><li>Shellfish</li><li>Red meat</li><li>Liver</li><li>Egg yolks</li><li>Cheese</li><li>Molasses</li><li>Brewer's yeast</li><li>Mushrooms</li><li>Whole wheat</li></ul>

As you can see from the actions of chromium listed above, it is a key nutrient in the combat of blood sugar control and diabetes. It can help to stabilise blood sugar levels through helping your body to use insulin more efficiently, and through calming sugar cravings.

Copper

Why do you need it?	Signs of possible deficiency	Where do you find it?
♋ Healthy bones and connective tissue ♋ Production of red blood cells ♋ Aids the absorption of iron ♋ Cardio vascular health ♋ Prevention of high blood pressure ♋ Protects against free radicals ♋ Protects against cancer	♋ Weakness ♋ Skin problems ♋ Breathing problems ** Deficiency is not common	♋ Offal ♋ Oysters ♋ Shellfish ♋ Whole grains ♋ Nuts ♋ Seeds ♋ Avocados ♋ Potatoes ♋ Garlic ♋ Bananas ♋ Mushrooms ♋ Cocoa ♋ Tomatoes ♋ Prunes ♋ Soya products

Iodine

Why do you need it?	Signs of possible deficiency	Where do you find it?
♋ Manufacture of hormones by the thyroid gland ♋ Regulation of metabolism ♋ Converting fats into energy ♋ Stabilising cholesterol levels	♋ Enlarged thyroid gland ♋ Dry skin ♋ Tiredness ** Deficiency is not common	♋ Table salt ♋ Seafood ♋ Saltwater fish ♋ Seaweed

Iron

Why do you need it?	Signs of possible deficiency	Where do you find it?
Carries oxygen around the body Needed to metabolise B vitamins Boosts immune function	Anaemia Tiredness Headaches / faintness Hair loss Digestive problems	Cockles Cocoa powder Molasses Soya produce Liver and kidney Dark green vegetables Dried fruit Egg yolk Shellfish Nuts

Magnesium

Why do you need it?	Signs of possible deficiency	Where do you find it?
Heart health Liver health Helps control good nerve & muscle function Balances metabolism Production and repair of cells Helps absorption of calcium PMS	Muscle fatigue Cramps Loss of appetite; nausea Numbness and tingling Eye tremors	Whole grains Nuts Millet Molasses Pulses / legumes Soya beans All green vegetables Shrimps & seafood

We use large amounts of magnesium, and need a regular supply. For example, over 300 of the enzymes that our bodies manufacture and require to carry our many of our bodily functions use and rely upon magnesium.

Absorption is aided by calcium, vitamin B6 and vitamin D.

Absorption is hindered by alcohol, caffeine, high levels of saturated fats, sugar and stress.

Manganese

Why do you need it?	Signs of possible deficiency	Where do you find it?
• Protection of the body's cells particularly against damage from free radicals • Metabolism and digestion • Helps to break down fats and cholesterol • Healthy bones and tissues	• Digestive problems • Dizziness • Loss of hearing	• Nuts • Brown rice • Cereals • Whole grains • Pulses / legumes

Molybdenum

Why do you need it?	Signs of possible deficiency	Where do you find it?
• Necessary for the production of DNA • Also known as an antioxidant • Helps to break down sulphites in foods, where if a toxic build-up occurs, it could lead to an allergic reaction • Prevention of tooth decay	• Breathing difficulties • Allergic reactions	• Liver • Whole grains • Yeast • Pulses / legumes • Leafy green vegetables

Phosphorus

Why do you need it?	Signs of possible deficiency	Where do you find it?
• Strong bones and teeth • Essential for energy production • Structural part of many cells	• Weak and painful bones • Weak teeth • Stiff joints • Tiredness ** Deficiency is not common	• Meat • Poultry • Fish • Dairy products • Nuts • Seeds • Whole grains

Because phosphorus is found in many processed foods, as a component of additives and preservatives (think phosphates!), a deficiency of this mineral is very rare in many parts of the world.

However, conversely, for those who consume a large proportion of processed foods, there can be an imbalance in which there is an excess of phosphorus. Another reason to eat good, fresh produce!

Potassium

Why do you need it?	Signs of possible deficiency	Where do you find it?
• Helps regulate fluid and acid/alkaline balance • Regulates heart rhythm • Transports oxygen to the brain • Key in enzyme production • Blood sugar control • Helps lower blood pressure	• Kidneys control the potassium / sodium balance in the body; if fails can lead to: • Irregular heart beat • Muscle aches and pains • Cramps • constipation • Depression and headaches • Confusion • Extreme thirst	• Vegetables • Fruit • Whole grains • Soya flour • Brown rice • Nuts and seeds • Molasses • Fish

Sustained exercise can lead to a depletion of potassium. A vital mineral, present in every cell in our bodies.

Selenium

This is a really interesting mineral, and as yet, the knowledge about selenium remains incomplete. It is not yet fully known what the consequences of a deficiency of selenium may be. However, it is known that in many cases of really serious illness, patients have very low levels of selenium. Whether it is the deficiency of selenium that causes these serious illnesses, or whether serious illnesses deplete the body of selenium, has yet to be identified!

Why do you need it?	Signs of possible deficiency	Where do you find it?
Good for healthy liver	Could lead to a higher risk of:	Nuts
Good for eyes		Molasses
Good for hair	Cancer	White fish
Good for nails	Heart disease	Liver and kidney
Good for skin	Skin problems	Shellfish
Helps regulate hormones		Whole grains
Protects from free-radical damage		Dairy products

Sodium

Why do you need it?	Signs of possible deficiency	Where do you find it?
Helps to maintain muscles	A deficiency is very rare but is possible through sweating, diarrhoea or vomiting and symptoms include:	Salt
Helps to maintain nerves		Shellfish
Works together with potassium to regulate fluids in the body		Anchovies
	Sickness	Dairy products especially butter
	Dizziness	Yeast extracts
	Muscle cramps	Processed meats
	Dehydration	Avocados
		Offal

Sulphur

Why do you need it?	Signs of possible deficiency	Where do you find it?
- An important component of several amino acids, which are needed to form proteins in the body - Detoxifying and eliminating any toxins from the body - May delay the ageing process - May delay the onset of any age-related diseases	- None are specifically identified.	- Meat - Poultry - Beans - Pulses / legumes - Shellfish

Zinc

Why do you need it?	Signs of possible deficiency	Where do you find it?
- Good for tissue repair - Wound healing - Healthy immune system - Digestive health - Reproductive health - Enzyme and insulin production	- Loss of smell and taste - Skin problems (acne and eczema) - Cuts that are slow to heal - Frequent colds - Disturbed sleep	- Seafood (oysters) - Popcorn - Nuts and seeds - Whole grains - Pulses / legumes - Sardines - Beef - Pork - Poultry - Ginger root - Green vegetables

By now you will definitely appreciate that consuming your full range of minerals really means having a varied and interesting diet, rich in great tasting fresh produce!

Antioxidants

There is a lot of talk about antioxidants, but what exactly are they? These are also nutrients about which our knowledge is still emerging – we don't yet know everything about antioxidants or their benefits to the human body. Here, I share what we do know.

First let me ask you a question...

When you bite into an apple and leave it, why does the flesh turn brown?

The answer is oxidation!

So what is oxidation? Well it's basically an interaction between oxygen and other substances. It occurs everywhere in nature, and results in unstable molecules called 'free radicals', which start chain reactions: apples turn brown, iron rusts, copper turns green/blue. In the human body the damage caused by oxidation can be severe. Called 'oxidative stress', it damages and even kills our living cells.

This is a bizarre dichotomy: we need oxygen to survive, but, at the same time, oxygen is killing our living cells, setting up disease conditions that eventually lead to our own deaths. Our bodies naturally produce enzymes to try to fight oxidative stress, preventing the damage that it chaotically causes. But, when oxidation occurs at high levels it overpowers our natural ability to prevent oxidative damage. That's when antioxidants can be helpful, but more about them in a while!

Research shows oxidative stress may contribute to:

- Alzheimer's disease
- Parkinson's disease
- rheumatoid arthritis
- neurodegeneration e.g. motor neuron diseases
- cardiovascular disease e.g. atherosclerosis
- oxidative damage in DNA that can cause cancer
- pathologies caused by diabetes

The latter of these of course is of especial interest to us in terms of helping us to combat diabetes and the complications that go with it.

Antioxidants are substances that may protect cells from the damage caused by free radicals. Our bodies maintain complex systems of multiple types of antioxidants, such as:

- glutathione
- vitamin C
- vitamin E
- enzymes such as catalase, superoxide dismutase and various peroxidases

Low levels of antioxidants, or inhibition of the antioxidant enzymes, are also associated with oxidative stress. That's because they fail to effectively deal with free radicals, which are fundamentally unstable because they have space in their chemical structure to bind with other molecules. Typically they bind with oxygen, which sets of a chain reaction within our cells that can lead to damage or even to the death of our affected cells. Because the free radicals bind with oxygen, they prevent our cells from using that oxygen in a normal healthy manner. Antioxidants, therefore, as their name suggests, prevent this binding with oxygen, known as oxidation, leaving the oxygen free and available to our cells.

Whilst our own bodies can make the antioxidants, listed above, for us, most are obtained from our diet from good plant-based foods.

Some vitamins, such as A, C, E, and minerals, such as selenium, act as antioxidants, but there are also other compounds and substances that behave in this antioxidant manner too. Examples are:

- **Flavonoids / polyphenols, found in:**
  - Soy
  - Red wine
  - Purple grapes
  - Pomegranate
  - Cranberries
  - Tea
  - Green tea
  - Onions
- **Lycopene, found in:**
  - Tomato and tomato products
  - Pink grapefruit
  - Watermelon
  - Berry fruits

- **Lutein, found in:**
  - Dark green vegetables such as kale, broccoli, brussels sprouts and spinach
  - Kiwi fruit
  - Corn
  - Cantaloupe
  - Butternut squash
  - Mango
- **Lignan, found in:**
  - Flax seeds / Linseeds
  - Oatmeal
  - Barley
  - Rye

You will probably recognise many of these foods that have become known as 'superfoods'. Well, this is why they are considered to be so super! They protect our bodies from damage at a cellular level, and in doing so help to prevent major illnesses in which cellular deterioration or even death plays a part.

Opinion about which are the best antioxidants varies: new superfoods are discovered ever more frequently it seems. It is best to remember, therefore, that antioxidants are found in abundance in beans, grain products, fruits and vegetables. Different antioxidants are associated with different colours in the vegetable world. Lutein tends to be found in yellow-pigmented plant foods, lycopene in red etc.

'the 6 diet' tells us that eating a fabulous variety of colourful vegetables is the way to go. Varied, interesting, tasty and even pretty! But all fresh, natural, unprocessed!!

Here is another note of caution: our limited knowledge of antioxidants means that it isn't absolutely certain how, or even if, antioxidants prevent disease. What we do know though is that consuming the foods that contain antioxidants is confirmed to benefit health! Which means that eating the foods rich in antioxidants is definitely better than taking antioxidant supplements: think tomato-based capsules containing high levels of lycopene, which have emerged into our health food shops in recent years! Indeed, highly potent supplements have been shown in some clinical trials to actually be damaging to health, therefore, it is much safer to obtain good antioxidants from natural foods!

Personalising your nutritional consumption

So far we have looked at some broad nutritional principles and information, which might enable anyone to adopt a much healthier diet. However **'the 6 diet'** is so much more than this. As I constantly say, there is no suitable one-size-fits-all dietary plan. You need, and deserve, a plan tailored precisely for your unique you!

With my Chinese medicine head on, I strongly recommend that you build in some Chinese dietetic principles too. Now please don't worry about this! You can still get massive benefit from **'the 6 diet'** without paying any attention to Chinese dietetics. However, I have come to know first-hand, for myself, and working with my patients, just how valuable this dietary paradigm can be. I would feel very remiss, therefore, if I didn't share it with you, so I hope you do read on. If you have trouble understanding this section that's OK – after all it contains concepts quite alien to most of us in the west. Maybe consult a traditional Chinese acupuncturist or Chinese medicine practitioner – they will certainly be able to point you at the bits of advice that can specifically help you!

The role for traditional Chinese dietetics

Traditional Chinese medicine, as the name suggests, originated in China many centuries ago. It was developed from close observations about the body, mind, spirit, disease and the effects of environment, lifestyle and diet on us. This form of medicine has only been practised in the west for a few decades and is increasing in popularity. This is testament to its effectiveness. Surely, no one would turn to this unfamiliar, ancient form of medicine unless it works? We are seeing more and more people seeking solutions in complementary and alternative forms of medicine, many of which are based on traditional Chinese medicine. These include acupuncture, Chinese herbal medicine, acupressure massage, shiatsu and other forms of energetic body work. Traditional Chinese medicine provides many valuable lessons about food and diet and their effects on our health and overall well-being. Practitioners of traditional Chinese therapies often provide dietary advice as part of their treatments.

We have talked already about the need to convert energy from our foods, and, in a modern nutritional sense, that great energy comes from digestion and metabolism of carbohydrates at a rate that matches our energetic needs.

There are clear parallels here with the traditional Chinese understanding of dietetics, in that success is all about energetic balance: BUT the understanding of what constitutes 'energy' is very different.

Different, that is, but not contradictory! Indeed, it is truly complementary.

By taking a view of energy in the round, combining the views of east and west, you create a powerful understanding of how to get the very best from your own body: in terms of appearance, performance, health.

Let's take a moment to look at the Chinese concept of energy:

Energy, or qi (pronounced chee) as it is in Chinese, is everything and everywhere. To avoid confusion between the two concepts of energy - western and eastern – we'll say 'energy' when we are talking from the western perspective, and 'qi' when from the Chinese perspective.

At its most simple level, traditional Chinese medicine is similarly about balancing qi in the body. When there is a deficiency of qi, or where qi becomes stagnant, pain, disease or disharmony develops. Where the qi flows smoothly and harmoniously this naturally creates well-being.

So how does food and diet play its part?

If we consider that qi is in everything, and everything is made of qi, then this also applies to our food.

In fact every food type is considered to have specific qi properties of its own. This means that specific foods may also be used to adjust the qi within our bodies - we have foods that are directly able to help move qi, build qi etc. Foods, therefore, may be used to influence the qi in the body in every way required to treat the multitude of conditions that respond to traditional Chinese therapies. Weight, appearance, body shape etc. are all outward manifestations of what happens internally within our bodies.

Diagnosis from a Chinese perspective is a complicated process, and it would be impossible to cover all aspects in this book. For now, however, there are some aspects of the nature of qi that need to be appreciated in order to be able to intelligently use the qi of food to our benefit.

When qi flows wrongly we may experience a range of symptoms. Some of the common imbalances that may arise are as follows:

- We may have a deficiency of qi and feel lethargic and unmotivated
- We may generate internal dampness – which is a particularly obstructive quality in our qi
- We may have a qi blockage (stagnation) or stasis of blood
- We may generate too much internal heat – giving rise to heat-related signs and symptoms within our bodies, or even emotionally
- We may generate too much internal cold – giving rise to cold-related signs and symptoms
- We may have a deficient cooling mechanism (subtly different from too much heat!)

- We may have a deficient warming mechanism (subtly different from too much cold!)
- Our qi may be unable to support our blood and other bodily substances

There are foods containing the qi properties to support our bodies and act as a remedy to the conditions above, bringing us back into a state of balance and bodily harmony: benefiting our appearance, health and vitality.

In the next few paragraphs we will explore each of these conditions in turn, and look at some of the ways they may arise, what effects they have on our bodies, and how foods may be used to counteract them.

About your qi

Qi deficiency

Most of us know very little about our spleen. We have no doubt heard of it, and might loosely understand that it has a role in the process of digestion. But still it tends to be one of the 'minor' organs that we take little notice of, except on the rare occasion when something goes wrong.

You may be very surprised to learn then, that in traditional Chinese medicine, the spleen is seen as the major digestive organ, with the stomach only playing a supporting role. Whilst we cannot ignore the stomach in terms of the digestive process (and we will discuss that later), at least according to the theory of traditional Chinese medicine, it is the spleen that requires your real attention.

It is the spleen's function to process the food and fluids that we eat and drink, and transform the pure nutrients to make qi. The qi generated by this transformation process is then transported around the body and used by all the other organs to maintain normal bodily functions for which they are collectively responsible.

When considering weight loss, health and vitality, the importance of the digestive system's ability to digest food properly and extract all the nutrients required to support our bodily functions is quite apparent. It is easy for us to understand the relevance or importance of this function. Also, because we can recognise similarities between this and the concept of digestion in orthodox medicine, we can readily accept the logic of this function. We already have a scientific understanding of the role that food plays in providing us with energy, and its contribution to good health.

When this function is not working properly we are most likely to feel tired and lethargic. In severe cases we may feel the fatigue at a spiritual level, having no interest in life, and probably no motivation to look after ourselves properly. This is because the body is not provided with good quality qi. The two parts of this function can contribute to this. Either food is not properly transformed to extract the qi, or the spleen fails to fulfil its purpose to transport the qi to other parts of the body, which consequently makes us feel fatigued.

According to traditional Chinese dietetics, there are foods with specific properties to help us to build great qi. These would be indicated and appropriate for anyone with a qi deficiency condition.

Internal dampness

When food is not properly transformed it accumulates in the body, giving rise to a condition called internal dampness.

It is this dampness that so often leads to an accumulation of excess body fat. Furthermore, it makes us feels heavy and sluggish. We may experience abdominal bloating or discomfort, perhaps even pain. This may affect our appetite, sometimes turning us off the idea of food. Think here of people you know who may be obviously overweight, but who cannot face breakfast for example. We may feel as though we are dragging heavy limbs around, or as though we are walking through treacle. Everything we do may feel slow and laboured.

As if that is not enough, we may even look damp. When the spleen function is efficient the flesh is toned and firm. It has a healthy glow and colour. However, when this function is not carried out properly, the flesh becomes flabby, puffy, dull and grey. Our complexions look lifeless, and unappealing. According to traditional Chinese medicine, overweight and obesity occur where there is a chronic accumulation of internal dampness. Rather poetically, it is considered that this internal dampness *floods into the flesh'*, resulting in excess body fat.

There may be many roots to the accumulation of internal dampness. In traditional Chinese medicine diagnosis is a complicated process, and internal dampness may occur as a result of many causes. Some are particularly relevant in overweight and obesity and need to be taken into account when trying to achieve weight loss or improved muscular tone. However, one thing remains true in all cases of overweight or obesity: where there is excess body fat, there is always the need to resolve internal dampness accumulated in the body.

Traditional Chinese dietetics classifies some foods as having damp qualities. For anyone experiencing the effects of internal dampness these foods would be contraindicated. On the other hand, some foods are able to help resolve internal dampness, and of course these would be especially appropriate to help overcome dampness problems.

Qi stagnation

Where qi is not circulated properly, it becomes stagnant. When this stagnation occurs in the meridians, we most often experience pain or other kinds of physical or emotional disharmony.

In relation to digestion there are two main causes. These are the two conditions we have just discussed:

- **The first is qi deficiency.**
  When there is a lack of qi to generate a smooth flow or circulation around the body small pockets of stagnation may occur. The analogy that I like to use here is that of a river in a hot dry climate: when the dry season advances, and the water in a river bed begins to recede and dry out it doesn't do so cleanly – instead pools or puddles of stagnant water begin to take the place of the flowing river before it becomes completely dry. In the same way, where qi is deficient, and a good steady flow cannot be maintained, it has a propensity to collect in small localised areas.
- **The second is internal dampness.**
  Being obstructive by nature, internal dampness hinders smooth qi flow, leading to its stagnation.

Some foods serve to move qi, so helping to resolve stagnation, and restore the smooth and harmonious flow of qi throughout the body.

At this point I should mention that the spleen is also responsible for other aspects of our health and well-being, but, so as not to become too technical or to cloud the picture, I have deliberately omitted to explain these additional functions in this book. I have included all you need to use **'the 6 diet'**!

A little later we'll take a close look at what damages our spleen's ability to carry out its functions, and what we can do to support and strengthen it.

Blood stasis

Just as qi may stagnate, blood flow may also become impaired, giving rise to a condition of blood stasis. Very often this goes hand in hand with qi stagnation, and indeed may arise as a result of qi stagnation, or it may be resultant of a blood deficiency in exactly the same way that qi stagnation may arise from qi deficiency.

Excess heat

The qi in our bodies can become too hot. This may occur for several reasons, and is usually recognisable by physical signs of heat, redness, dryness etc. Emotionally, too much heat might lead to irritability or even bigger emotional outbursts – just think about the tetchiness that you might feel on a really hot summer's day when you cannot cool down and the links between internal heat and temper become clear.

Digestively, internal heat becomes like an inner fire that demands to be stoked. A typical symptom of internal heat might, therefore, be an insistent hunger - one that isn't satisfied for long after eating. There is a rather lovely east-west cross-over here: think of the lack of satiety caused by eating excessive amounts of sugar. We have already discussed, in previous chapters, the blood-sugar consequences of consuming a diet high in sugars or refined carbohydrate foods. The resultant peaks and troughs in our blood glucose levels cause us to quickly hunger again, even though it may only be a short time since eating.

Some foods are energetically heating by nature, and some are cooling. When a body is too hot, and frequently hungers, it demands food in just the same way as when there is a really poor blood-sugar balance.

It is essential, to encourage the body back to a state of thermal balance, to avoid foods with a heating nature, and to emphasise foods with a cooling nature.

Excess cold

The flip side of the coin is that the qi in our bodies can become too cold. Again, this may occur for several reasons, but it is usually recognisable by physical signs of cold or chilliness. In order to bring the body back into thermal balance, the importance is on the emphasis of warming foods and an avoidance of cooling foods which would further exacerbate the problem.

Think how comforting and nourishing a great soup, stew or casserole is in the winter time, and how ice-cream simply isn't too appealing!

Deficiency in cooling

Our bodies have an innate cooling mechanism. In Chinese medicine, cooling is seen as a role for our Yin qi. If our yin becomes deficient then our bodies may begin to develop signs of heat. It can be really tricky to differentiate excessive heat from a deficient cooling mechanism, because general signs of heat will occur in each scenario.

'the 6 diet' provides the tools to make this differentiation for you: if you decide not to follow the system then I would strongly urge you to make an appointment for a professional practitioner of Chinese medicine to help you to make sense of your own signs and symptoms of heat.

Whilst there is still some sense in avoiding heating foods and making a special effort to eat cooling foods, there is even more sense in getting right to the bottom of the issue, and eating those foods that will also support your body's own Yin qi.

Deficiency in warming

Our bodies have an innate warming mechanism. In Chinese medicine, warming is seen as a role for our Yang qi. If our yang becomes deficient then our bodies may begin to develop signs of cold. Just as in the case of excess heat vs. deficient cooling, it can be really tricky to differentiate excessive cold from a deficient warming mechanism, because signs of cold will occur in each scenario.

Again, **'the 6 diet'** provides the tools to make this differentiation for you: or use the services of a professional practitioner of traditional Chinese medicine to help you to make sense of your own signs and symptoms of cold.

Just as some foods can help to support our yin qi, and hence our bodies' abilities to cool, there are also those foods that can help to support our yang qi. These will stoke our own abilities to maintain and appropriate physiological warmth.

Supporting blood

As well as using nutrition to generate great qi, our bodies also need to constantly generate blood and other bodily substances. Some circumstances mean that our ability to do just that, or at least to generate enough, is impaired or compromised. Some foods have the properties to support good blood formation.

I am often asked whether a deficient blood condition is the same as anaemia. It can be similar, but is not identical: though it's a good parallel to illustrate the point that we do need to support our blood production through foods! Just as in a case involving anaemia we may emphasise the importance of iron-rich foods, in the Chinese medicine sense we may have a need to emphasise good blood-forming foods.

You'll need capable resources in order to determine for yourself whether or not you have a particular need to emphasise those blood forming foods within your own diet. **'the 6 diet'**, or a professional practitioner of traditional Chinese medicine, will help you to make sense of your own bodily needs.

It's worth investing a little time and some resources into exploring your nutritional needs from a traditional Chinese dietetics perspective. The level of precision that you could bring to bear for the benefit of your own body is unparalleled. Here's a great example of what this means:

> *"There are two people suffering from arthritis, one experiencing hot, painful joints, and the other experiencing a worsening of their symptoms in cold, damp weather. According to our modern nutritional understanding we may advise oily fish as beneficial for joint health for both individuals: great essential fatty acids, and especially Omega-3! Some of the most commonly available types of oily fish include tuna, salmon, mackerel, sardines, trout. These have very different properties according to traditional Chinese dietetics, especially in terms of their thermal energetics: several are considered neutral, whilst salmon is cooling and trout is warming. This means that salmon may be especially beneficial for the person experiencing hot, painful arthritis, and trout advisable for the one whose symptoms are aggravated by cold."*

'the 6 diet' is the only nutritional approach that combines the best from both Western and Chinese dietary paradigms for your benefit, and I know from my own nutritional journey just how valuable it really is to consider both aspects.

It is my own experience of traditional Chinese dietetics (though I didn't know that was what it was at the time!) that gives me the absolute conviction of its value: try it and find out for yourself.

Let me share my own personal story with you:

A Personal Journey Towards Food Enlightenment!

About 20 years ago I caught a virus. This was actually the start of the journey that ultimately led me to study the material that I have used to formulate the advice for you contained within **'the 6 diet'**

There is little treatment available for viral infections, and medical tests showed that it would take about 2 years for my recovery to be completed. In itself it caused few obvious problems. But, when your immune system fights a long-term virus it can leave the body more open to bacterial infection. For many months I contracted one respiratory infection after another. I had many nasty 'itises' and all the antibiotics to go with them! The implications of long-term use of antibiotics is better known now, but back then I was given no advice or protection from killing off my 'good bacteria'. In the end my treatment left me with a condition called systemic candida. In other words, the yeasts that live naturally in our gut, and are normally controlled by the good bacteria, had rampaged out of control. I was left with a chronic fatigue, lots of additional body fat, and had no energy at all. I was very fortunate to have a kinesiologist friend who recognised my condition, carried out food tolerance tests and prescribed me a restricted diet. Under her advice, I steered clear of certain types of food and very quickly began to feel much better. For about 18 months I stuck rigidly to my food regime, and was amazed, and delighted, to find that not only did I regain health, I lost almost 2 stones in weight. This was despite eating heartily of the foods that I was allowed!

It wasn't until I started to study traditional Chinese medicine a few years later that I realised that my diet was extremely closely aligned with the concepts of energy balancing. It took no convincing me that the dietary regime advocated by the Chinese would certainly lead to weight-loss, great health and vitality. I already had the personal evidence.

I urge you to take advantage of these great principles for yourself.

Elaine x

In this next section, we'll look at some general advice about how to look after your digestive qi, to enable you make the very best of your food, and your body! Regardless of your starting point, in terms of weight and health, looking after your digestive system is key to improved bodily appearance and performance.

Looking after your spleen qi

The role of the spleen

The spleen is one of the major organs according to Chinese medicine. It has several functions that are quite challenging concepts for anyone unschooled in traditional Chinese medicine. I'll try to explain as simply as I can, but in turn you'll maybe have to suspend everything you may already know about this oft-neglected organ.

Transformation of Food and Transportation of Qi

We have already touched on this as one of the major functions of the spleen. It processes the food and fluids that we eat and drink, and uses the pure nutrients to make qi. The qi that is produced from this transformation process is then transported around the body, and used by all the other organs and tissues to maintain the normal bodily functions for which they are collectively responsible.

When food is not properly transformed it accumulates in the body, often giving rise to the condition of internal dampness as discussed earlier.

We have already looked at the consequences of internal dampness: excess body fat; feelings of heaviness and sluggishness; abdominal bloating or discomfort; perhaps even pain; abnormal appetite; feeling as though we are dragging heavy limbs around; feeling as though we are walking through treacle; a grey, pasty and puffy complexion.

All physically and aesthetically unappealing indeed!

Raising Qi

The normal flow of qi from the spleen takes place in an upward direction. Thus, the spleen is said to be responsible for raising qi in the body. This helps us to hold ourselves erect. It holds our organs in their proper place inside the body. When functioning efficiently, therefore, the spleen prevents the prolapse of organs. Also it assists the upward movement of the circulation of blood returning to the heart from the lower parts of the body.

When this function is impaired, and the spleen is unable to fulfil its responsibility to raise qi, a variety of medical complaints may be apparent. These might include the prolapse of organs, such as the uterus, bladder, or anus – the latter causing us to experience haemorrhoids. If the blood in the legs does not efficiently return to the heart we may develop varicose veins. In less severe cases we may simply experience the sensation of heaviness, as described above, more in our lower body and limbs.

With regards to overweight and obesity, it is the impairment of this function that can be considered to be responsible for the pear-shaped silhouette that we are so familiar with in the west. This is simply a matter of the excess body fat settling on the lower parts of the body, i.e. the hips and thighs, as a result of the qi sinking along with the naturally heavier dampness.

Maintaining Clear Thinking

On the face of it, this function is probably a little more difficult for us to understand. In essence, the spleen is responsible for maintaining the capacity for clear thinking. It is closely linked with raising qi. By raising pure qi to the head, the spleen creates the conditions for clarity of thinking. The raising of pure qi to the head replaces the older, less pure qi, which is responsible for muddied thinking.

When this function works efficiently we are able to see our way clearly through everyday situations, even problems. We are able to be creative in finding ways to meet normal day-to-day challenges and to be able to solve trickier problems. When faced with change we are able to adapt readily. This affects our ability to cope on a practical level, and also to grasp new intellectual ideas. After all, we talk about 'brain foods', such as fish, some vegetables etc., so we already have an understanding at some level that food does affect our capacity to think.

When the spleen is impaired, and fails to carry out this function efficiently, we find it difficult to think properly. This does not just affect our capacity to work out solutions to complicated problems, or to solve intellectual puzzles. It also means that we often cannot see our way past every day issues. How many times have you found yourself unable to sleep at night, as mundane thoughts fill your brain, refusing to move to allow sleep to take place? This pattern of circular thinking is most commonly associated with the spleen. It shows a real stuckness in thinking, and is very often characterised by the 'yes, but...' pattern of thinking.

Perhaps you recognise that you think way about your ability to make real changes to benefit yourself both in terms of your appearance or your health (or both!)? If so, I would urge you to read on!

Governing Flesh

This function is very closely linked to the function of transporting qi throughout the body. Where qi is not circulated properly, it becomes stagnant. When this stagnation occurs in the meridians, we most often experience pain. But when that stagnation occurs in the flesh, internal dampness is deposited by the qi, which is unable to move smoothly. The dampness accumulates, and we become fat. This is the unfortunate reality of the poetic Chinese notion of internal dampness flooding the flesh to cause overweight and obesity.

When this function is efficient the flesh is toned and firm. It has a healthy glow and colour. However, when this function is not carried out properly, the flesh becomes flabby, puffy, dull and grey.

What harms your spleen?

OK, so now we know a little bit about what the spleen does for us. Hopefully you now have a motivation to take care of your spleen? There are some don'ts and some dos! The following paragraphs outline those habits and practices that may be harmful to your spleen's ability to care for your qi:

Damp Foods and Conditions

In traditional Chinese medicine, it is often true to say that what goes around comes around. Causes become effects and effects become causes. So just as an unhealthy spleen will cause an accumulation of internal dampness, so dampness introduced into the body will cause the spleen qi to become unhealthy. Such dampness may enter the body via the food that we consume, or from the environment. Living, working or playing in damp conditions may eventually deplete the spleen. However, as you can imagine, one of the most common causes of spleen deficiency is the consumption of energetically damp foods. By now you are probably coming to understand that a 'damp' diet is the most common cause of overweight and obesity. The single most important thing we can do for ourselves if we want to lose weight, or to promote our spleen's ability to take care of us, is to avoid energetically damp foods. It is important at this point to understand that when we talk about dampness in foods, we are referring to the energetic properties of the food, and not necessarily the fact that it is damp or wet to touch.

A list of those foods that are considered to be dampening is provided a little later.

Excess Raw and Cold Foods

The spleen does not take kindly to an excessive consumption of raw or cold foods. When we refer to cold foods, in this context, we are talking both about the temperature of food, and the energetic properties of the foods. Too much chilled food and drink inhibit the normal functioning of the spleen. Similarly foods having energetically cold qualities also inhibit spleen function.

This really flies in the face of some of our modern ideas about food – we so often have a notion that salads and fruit are good for us. Well hopefully **'the 6 diet'** has sufficiently convinced us, from a modern scientific perspective, that an excessive intake of fruit is simply too sugary and disturbs our blood sugar balance – leading to all the consequences that are associated with that! It should give us some faith in the traditional Chinese dietetic approach to know that this has been recognised for millennia!

But raw food? Well, yes!

The very latest clinical research into the consumption of raw foods versus their cooked counterparts shows that the nutrients in cooked foods tend to be more easily absorbed by our bodies than those from raw foods. Whilst it is true that the raw food contains more nutrients overall than the cooked ones, you may be surprised to learn that after eating them you will benefit from more nutrients finding their way into your bloodstream from the cooked foods than from the raw. This is another piece of **'the 6 diet'** jigsaw that may be new to our modern nutritional understanding, but which the Chinese have long embraced.

Long-term overuse of raw and cold foods leads to spleen deficiency, so resulting in the now familiar pattern of internal damp accumulation and subsequent body fat. When trying to lose weight, or simply to optimise digestive health, it is the avoidance of damp food that remains the priority, but nonetheless, it is necessary to watch the consumption of raw and cold foods.

Certainly, limiting ourselves to cold salads, raw fruits and vegetables, cold shakes, juices etc. is not the most effective way to benefit our bodies, yet, in western cultures, we often embark on such courses of action when attempting to eat healthily.

Too Much Food

In order to transform foods efficiently, the qi in the spleen organ needs to be able to flow and circulate freely. Just as overloading a washing machine prevents the water from circulating properly, and clothes remain dirty or unrinsed, when the smooth flow of spleen qi is impaired or blocked, the process of transformation is seriously hindered.

The advice of traditional Chinese dietetics, is to stop eating when you are 70% full. This may be sound advice, but begs the question, *'How do I know when I am 70% full?'* There is certainly no easy answer to this. But I hope that as you learn to recognise what happens within your own body and to your own energy after consuming different kinds and quantities of food this may become a little more intuitive. Suffice to say, at this stage, that it is wise to stop eating before you feel full, but do not stop eating when you are still experiencing hunger. There is some scientific basis, within our own medical understanding, for this advice – remember our friend leptin, and its role in helping us to regulate our appetites? It is known that the messages between the stomach and brain are quite slow to detect a cessation of hunger. Therefore, by carrying on eating until you no longer feel hungry, you have already passed the point at which you have taken in sufficient food to satisfy the brain anyway. By eating until you actually feel full means that you have really overeaten, probably giving rise to quite considerable discomfort for some time after your meal. Sounds familiar? I am sure we've all done this at some time or other, and have probably vowed never to do it again. **'the 6 diet'** tells us why this is actually harmful rather than simply uncomfortable!

Excess Fluids

The spleen does not like excess fluid. When eating a meal, the spleen is unable to carry out its functions of transformation and transportation efficiently where too much fluid is consumed. It is best to drink plenty of fluids, especially water, between meals. There are, again, parallels here with our modern understanding of the science of digestion. **'the 6 diet'** tells us that drinking too much whilst trying to digest food dilutes our stomach acid, preventing it from being able to properly act upon the food to break it down ready for the enzymatic part of digestion that takes place within the small intestine.

Irregular Dietary Habits

Skipping meals, eating at irregular hours, or eating on the go are all detrimental. With **'the 6 diet'** we understand why this is absolutely correct, considering the effects that dietary irregularity has in terms of blood-sugar balance, diabetes and its consequences!

Even where the diet is otherwise beneficial to the spleen, irregular dietary habits hinder the capacity of the spleen to function normally. This is certainly an example of how our lifestyle contributes to the increasing incidence of overweight and obesity in many cultures. Eating in a hurry is also contraindicated. The spleen needs time and space in which to execute its functions properly. It makes sense too, from a purely scientific perspective, that if there is a time lag between eating and the brain recognising the cessation of hunger, then the slower we eat, the less likely we are to over indulge, and overburden the digestive system as discussed above.

Excessive Thinking / Mental Overexertion

Again, it can be said that what goes around comes around. Whilst, as we have discussed previously, an unhealthy spleen can prevent clear thinking, so over-thinking taxes the spleen, leading to a deficiency of the spleen qi. Typically, this understanding is associated with excessive studying, but equally applies to any other form of mental exertion. Occupations requiring lots of thinking, problem solving, deliberations also tax the spleen, inhibiting its capacity to function effectively and efficiently.

This can establish a vicious cycle, in which the occupational need for over-thinking leads to an inability to think clearly. No wonder then that so many students and people employed in sedentary office jobs put on weight so easily. It is not simply a matter of lack of exercise, but according to traditional Chinese dietetics, an implication of the very type of work being undertaken. Couple this with an inappropriate diet, irregular eating patterns, eating on the go, or skipping meals, and the spleen is undoubtedly hit with a double whammy. Can you imagine the level of damage you might bring to bear by eating at your desk, or while watching the television, doing the crossword etc.?

'the 6 diet' tells us that there are scientific parallels here too: in later chapters we will discuss the role of stress on our digestive abilities and its consequences in terms of our bodily appearance, diabetes and general health.

What helps your spleen?

Simplistically, just about the exact opposite of what it dislikes is considered to be beneficial to the energetic spleen.

Warm Dry Foods and Conditions

The spleen prefers warming foods. This is again both in terms of thermal properties and energetic properties. This means that soups, broths and warming casseroles are much more suitable than the usual 'diet' foods, for nourishing and tonifying the spleen qi, encouraging its return to normal healthy functioning. Ideally the spleen prefers drier baked foods, though it is not essential to restrict the diet exclusively to these. Whilst, as we have said, cold, raw foods can lead to or exacerbate spleen qi deficiency, the watchword is to 'avoid' these foods. They are not quite so damaging to the spleen as damp foods, and if used in moderation and with care are not totally disastrous for most people. This is especially true if combined with the warm, dry, baked foods preferred by the spleen. For example, a salad can be tolerated if served as a side dish with a warm, cooked meal which is especially nourishing to the spleen.

A Regular and Relaxed Eating Pattern

Of course, if irregular dietary habits are considered damaging to the spleen, then the opposite is considered beneficial. Regular meal times are preferable. The best times of day for digesting food are discussed later, but it is sufficient for now to think about eating at regular intervals and not skipping meals. Remember, balancing food energies is much more about eating the right kinds of foods, balancing the type of qi consumed with the needs of the body. The quantities of food, in terms of calories etc. are less important, and so there is no gain when trying to lose weight in skipping meals or limiting quantities to starvation rations.

Also, the Chinese consider that the act of eating should be undertaken in a contemplative manner.

"When you walk, just walk
When you eat, just eat."
- Attributed to Buddha

This means clearing the mind, and concentrating, in a quiet and relaxed manner, on the task in hand. That is eating. Thus, the spleen is not burdened by over-thinking, or mental exertion, and is able to carry out its function of transformation and transportation more effectively. Of course, eating in quiet contemplation also requires us to refrain from reading or watching television when consuming food. Essentially eating whilst pursuing these activities is no different from eating on the run, as they still require us to apply our minds and thoughts to things other than the food we are eating and the act of eating itself.

Emotional and Spiritual Nourishment

Traditional Chinese philosophies, including medicine, Feng Shui etc., consider that there are five elements. These are Fire, Earth, Metal, Wood and Water. Each element governs an aspect of qi, be it qi within the environment or our bodies. We may already be familiar with the concepts of similar elements in terms of astrology, the zodiac, horoscopes etc.

The spleen is associated with the earth element. The earth element is aligned to nourishment on all levels, physical, emotional and spiritual. We may perceive this idea as we do mother earth, or mother nature. As such, the spleen likes nothing better than love and nurturing. This of course is something we can provide for ourselves, and does not require another person to provide these conditions for us. Indeed we all have a responsibility to take care of ourselves emotionally and spiritually as well as physically.

Later in this book we will cover more about this form of nourishment, and how to obtain it for ourselves. It is still worth mentioning here though that traditional Chinese medicine tells us that only about 25% of the spleen's nourishment is obtained from the foods and drink that we consume. That leaves a huge deficit of 75% to be sought elsewhere, indicating the great value that emotional and spiritual nourishment has in terms of ensuring a healthy energetic spleen, with sufficient capacity to fulfil its functions effectively and efficiently.

So, what about the stomach?

The role of the stomach

So, I did say that the stomach also has its part to play in digestion from a traditional Chinese medicine perspective. It is essentially a supporting role, but nonetheless it is important to consider the likes and dislikes of the stomach too in order to optimise your digestive ability.

From the perspective of Western scientific medicine, while most of us know very little about our spleen, we tend to be much more familiar with our stomach. Indeed, we probably consider the stomach to be the primary organ in the digestive system. As such, where digestive illnesses occur, we tend to talk about our 'stomach problems', almost regardless of where the real problems actually lie.

Therefore, in considering the role of the energetic stomach, we first need to suspend our scientific understanding about this organ, and again open our hearts and minds to the alternative theory underpinning traditional Chinese medicine.

Controls Rotting and Ripening of Food

This is one of the major functions of the stomach. Again, the language used to describe this function is typically poetic, but does, however, describe this function well. Essentially it describes the function by which the stomach prepares the food and fluids that we eat and drink, in readiness for the spleen to separate the pure nutrients from the waste and to extract the qi.

We can easily see that this function is very closely aligned with our own scientific knowledge about the functions of the stomach, and is therefore readily acceptable to us whatever our cultural background. Stomach acids and digestive enzymes are indeed responsible for breaking down the foods that we consume to enable us to extract and absorb the nutrients contained within. Similarly, in traditional Chinese medicine, it is recognised that the stomach needs fluids in order to carry out this function efficiently and effectively.

When this function is not working properly food is not broken down sufficiently to enable the spleen to transform the end product of the rotting and ripening process – an absolute parallel with the scientific understanding of the role for the stomach. When our stomachs do not function correctly we retain semi-rotted and semi-ripened foods and we experience this retention in a number of ways. We may feel full in and around the midriff or, to give it its more correct name, the epigastrium. This, of course, corresponds closely with the anatomical position of the stomach. In more severe cases the semi-processed food may travel backwards along the digestive tract. This upwards movement manifests as hiccups, belching, regurgitation, heartburn, indigestion, nausea or even vomiting. All are signs that the stomach energy is impaired, and failing to fulfil its normal function – and are exactly what we might experience from a modern perspective on having insufficient stomach acid. Of course, whenever this upward movement occurs we often experience a sour or rotten taste.

When food is not properly rotted and ripened, the spleen is unable to transform it. Where the spleen is unable to fulfil its own functions, any untransformed food accumulates in the body, giving rise to the condition of internal dampness. So, although it is not the primary digestive organ, the stomach still plays a vital role in maintaining good health and well-being, and of course a healthy body weight.

This is a good example of the supporting role played by the stomach. Where the stomach qi is impaired, and the stomach cannot function effectively, there is a direct knock on effect to the spleen, which in turn cannot carry out its own function properly.

Transportation of Qi

The stomach also supports the spleen function of transportation of qi around the body. The normal flow of qi from the stomach takes place in a downward direction. Thus, the stomach is said to be responsible for descending qi in the body.

When this function is impaired, the stomach is unable to fulfil its responsibility to descend qi and it becomes stuck or stagnant in the stomach. Where qi stagnates, heat may be generated. Rather like a pressure cooker, when the steam cannot escape from the cooker, it generates extremely high temperatures inside. Similarly, when the stomach qi stagnates it generates heat. This may be felt as heat in the stomach or upper digestive tract, in the form of burning pain. The traditional Chinese medicine diagnosis for peptic ulceration is poetically termed as 'stomach fire'. I guess anyone who has ever experienced the pain from a peptic ulcer might confirm that this is indeed a very accurate description!

Where the body senses this extreme heat, it calls for us to put out the fire. We feel this as hunger. Therefore, one of the symptoms of stomach heat or fire is a constant hunger. Of course the body is calling for cooling foods to counteract the heat, but if we are not aware of this we often choose the wrong foods, and simply end up stoking the fire, leading to further hunger. Individuals do not need to have peptic ulceration to feel this effect. Certainly, not every case of stomach heat or fire will result in an actual ulcer. However, for those who do suffer, it is often the case that the pain from an ulcer is temporarily soothed by food. Often the food that helps in this condition is milk, or other dairy products. Since these foods are energetically dampening, it is not difficult to see how they work. What better to pour over a fire than something damp! However, where the fire is stronger than the damp food the fire flares again and the pain returns a short time later.

If we again consider our pressure cooker analogy, when the weight is released from the lid, the steam escapes very quickly, forming a fast, hot upward jet. Again, we can compare this with the action of hot stomach qi, which also rises through the energy channel associated with the stomach. Because this movement is opposite to the normal flow of stomach qi it is described as counter-flow or rebellion of qi. The speed and violence of the rebellion determines the physical effect that we experience, from the less severe hiccups and belching, through to regurgitation, heartburn, indigestion, nausea and vomiting as mentioned above.

Furthermore, when stomach qi 'rebels', and flows upwards instead of downwards, an excess of hot stomach qi flows upward through the channel and, because of its anatomical route, can affect the face. We may experience this as a sour taste in the mouth, bad breath or halitosis, bleeding gums, or even toothache.

When heat enters the head, displacing the pure qi that the spleen normally raises, headaches may occur. It is often via this route that we can relate migraine attacks with certain foods. In more severe cases mental-emotional problems may arise. These are usually the more manic type of mental-emotional conditions characterised by sharp temper or violent outbursts. It is probably no coincidence that we refer to this as 'hot-headed' behaviour!

However, I must stress at this stage that nobody, unless properly trained and qualified in traditional

Chinese medicine should attempt to diagnose mental-emotional problems. This is an extremely complex area in which there are many possible diagnoses, most not involving the stomach energy at all! If you have any concerns about mental-emotional illnesses the only sensible course of action is to consult with an appropriate professional practitioner.

Descending Waste to the Small Intestine

This function is very closely linked to the function of descending qi through the body. Once the spleen has completed the process of transformation and transportation, the stomach is responsible for descending the waste into the small intestine.

When this function is efficient we experience smooth and regular bowel movements. However, when it is impaired we may experience either diarrhoea or constipation. I'm afraid it's time to get a little lavatorial! Diarrhoea may occur when the stomach and spleen energies are both too weak to carry out their respective functions properly. This kind of diarrhoea is often characterised by the presence of undigested foods. Where the spleen is damp but the stomach is hot, the diarrhoea may be hot, causing a burning sensation in the anus during the bowel movement. Constipation may occur when the stomach does not descend the waste efficiently, and there is nothing descended into the small intestine to form stools to be passed. Alternatively, stomach heat may dry out the waste products before they are descended to the small intestine. In such cases, the stools are very hard and dried and are very difficult to pass out in defecation.

What harms your stomach?

Taking care of the stomach, as well as the spleen, therefore makes perfect sense. Just as your spleen has its likes and dislikes, so does your stomach. In the next few paragraphs we'll look at the don'ts and the dos to benefit your stomach.

Excess Hot Foods & Conditions

Once again, in traditional Chinese medicine, we find that what goes around comes around. Causes become effects and effects become causes. So, just as an unhealthy stomach will give rise to heat or fire, external heat put into the body will impair the stomach qi. Given its capacity to generate extreme internal heat, almost the last thing the stomach can tolerate is excess external heat, either in the form of food, or from the environment.

Many hot-tasting spices, as shown later in our list of heating foods, also have hot energetic properties. So, as an example, let us consider how an otherwise normal healthy stomach reacts to a meal, such as curry, consisting of large quantities of hot spices. Even while eating such a meal we will likely feel physically hot. As the heat from the stomach begins to rise up through its associated meridian we may begin to feel heat in the head and face. We may begin to perspire on the forehead and face, and our complexion may even begin to look quite rosy and glowing. Our mouths will begin to burn. We may even begin to feel the heat in the epigastric region around the stomach itself. Belching soon after such a meal is commonplace. Later we may experience a 'stomach upset'. This may involve heartburn or indigestion, caused as the stomach heat rises through the digestive tract. Often we have a nauseating hollow feeling of hunger in our stomach, characterising the body's call for cool food to quench the heat or fire. Finally we may experience a hot, burning bowel movement. And all this, remember, in a fairly normal healthy stomach. This extreme picture also illustrates what can happen with less extreme foods in a stomach impaired by the presence of chronic internal heat or fire.

External environmental heat can also affect the digestive process. Therefore, we may find similar reactions also arise when we place ourselves in a hot climate. It is a common experience for many to find themselves struggling to combat constipation when holidaying in hot climes!

The drying effect of heat further explains its capacity to impair the energetic stomach. Internal heat dries out and desiccates stomach fluids, which are required to enable the stomach to fulfil its functions properly. More is said about the effects of dried stomach fluids below.

Excess of Extremely Cold Foods

The stomach is, perhaps contrarily, also unable to tolerate an excess of extremely cold foods. The reaction to extremely cold or chilled foods may be acute or chronic. That is to say it may be a sudden and violent reaction to an extremely cold food, or it may come on more slowly as a result of longer-term use of excessive cold foods. In its acute state, cold stomach qi is most commonly characterised by severe, violent, and often immediate rebellion of stomach qi. A good example of this is the sudden projectile vomiting that a small child may experience after eating an excessive amount of ice cream! In its more chronic state, cold stomach qi is recognisable by watery diarrhoea, often containing undigested foods; epigastric discomfort or pain together with a sense of chilliness and coldness to the touch; borborygmus, which is a noisy gurgling or rumbling stomach; and belching, indigestion or nausea.

The main way to spot the difference between the effects of cold on the stomach and spleen is that with the stomach, the signs and symptoms are more related to the midriff or epigastrium and include the upward flow of qi giving rise to indigestion, nausea etc.; whereas, with the spleen the signs and symptoms are more related to the abdomen. Of course, as both the stomach and spleen can be damaged by cold, it is likely that signs and symptoms of both will occur together anyway. This indicates the close supportive relationship between the two organs according to traditional Chinese medicine theory.

Excessive Dryness

As explained previously, sufficient stomach fluids are necessary to enable the function of rotting and ripening food. In this, we can see there is a common understanding between traditional Chinese medicine and our own scientific-based western medicine.

Where there is an excessive consumption of dry foods, or, more commonly, a lack of fluid intake, the stomach fluids dry out, and prevent the stomach from properly fulfilling its functions.

Similarly, an excessively dry climate can similarly affect the stomach. In this instance, excessive environmental dryness refers to little short of desert conditions.

Excessive Thinking / Mental Overexertion

The stomach, in common with the spleen, is also adversely affected by strenuous thinking and mental overexertion. This reflects the close relationship between the two organs, and as such requires little further explanation. Everything that we discussed earlier in relation to the effects of excessive mental activity on the spleen also apply to the stomach.

What helps your stomach?

Again, simplistically, just about the exact opposite of what the stomach dislikes is considered to be to its benefit. In addition, the stomach usefully shares some of its preferences with the spleen.

Cool, Moist Foods and Conditions

Because of its propensity to be affected by heat, it is perhaps no surprise to find that the stomach prefers cool, moist foods and environmental conditions. However, it is important to strike a balance when choosing cooling foods, taking care to ensure that foods and drinks are not too chilled, or at least limiting the amount of very cold or chilled food and drink. As we have discussed, the stomach does not tolerate extreme cold any more than heat, and the spleen also dislikes excessively cold foods and drinks.

Moderation is the key to maintaining healthy stomach qi. Therefore to benefit the stomach, it is advisable to incorporate gently cooling foods into the diet, except where signs of cold already exist.

Fluids, taken in the form of drinks, are needed to support the stomach fluids, which are essential to enable the stomach to properly rot and ripen foods. Again, the healthy stomach will have a preference for cooling fluids. However, care should be taken to avoid over-cooling the stomach qi, and certainly where signs of cold stomach qi already exist. In terms of the volume of fluid intake, it is essential to the healthy energetic functioning of the stomach to ensure that sufficient fluids are consumed, and that the body is not allowed to dehydrate. Where there are insufficient stomach fluids, and the function of rotting and ripening is impaired, the spleen will be unable to properly transform the foods to extract good quality qi, leading to the, now familiar, pattern of damp accumulation.

Of course, you probably now already understand this to be vitally important in achieving weight loss as well as good digestive health. Scientifically, **'the 6 diet'** has already described how when the body starts to become dehydrated, it tries to hold onto whatever internal fluid it has. Usually, the fluids that it retains are those trapped in the body tissues. Instead of constantly replenishing the tissue fluids, bathing them in fresh water, the trapped water becomes stagnant, and we feel and look sluggish and bloated. We usually recognise this as the condition we term 'water retention'. However, in its more serious form, water retention may become oedema. Commonly our feet and ankles, fingers and hands visibly swell to much larger proportions, and feel tight and hard. We also know that when we place ourselves in hotter climates we need to take special care to avoid dehydration by increasing our normal fluid intake.

A Regular and Relaxed Eating Pattern

In common with the spleen, and again as evidence of the close relationship between the two organs, the stomach also prefers dietary regularity. This means adopting fairly regular mealtimes and avoiding skipping meals, to establish a supportive eating pattern.

Also, as with the spleen, the stomach prefers a relaxed, contemplative approach to eating. This means sitting down quietly to eat without distraction. Eating on the go, or eating hurriedly is to be avoided. Again, as we discussed when looking at the energetic spleen, it is also beneficial for the stomach is we avoid reading, watching TV, or engaging in any other mental activity when eating.

Emotional and Spiritual Nourishment

The stomach is also associated with the earth element, which as we have previously said, is aligned to nourishment on all levels, physical, emotional and spiritual. This means that by involving ourselves with activities or practices that calm our minds and provide emotional and spiritual nourishment we optimise the body's ability to fulfil its digestive function efficiently and effectively.

We have more about this to follow later!

Traditional Chinese medicine view of diabetes

Traditional Chinese medicine is able to explain any illness or disease from the perspective of what it calls 'patterns'. Being a holistic paradigm means that, unlike in Western medicine, it focuses not on a single sign or symptom, such as too much glucose in the blood, but on an overall presentation of collections of signs and symptoms. Of course having too much glucose in the blood stream is just one presenting sign that must be taken into account alongside many others that any individual might present with or experience. For example, signs that an individual may have diabetes include frequent urination, abnormal thirst, slow healing of wounds, unexplained weight loss, dry or itchy skin, abnormal hunger or fatigue, and numbness in the feet. Whilst different people may experience any combination, or maybe all, of these signs and symptoms, in western medicine they will all be given the same diagnosis: diabetes. However, these different indications may point to different patterns in a traditional Chinese medicine sense. In this way two people with diabetes might be diagnosed as having quite different patterns in terms of traditional Chinese medicine.

That said, there are several patterns that commonly occur in people presenting with diabetes. These include blood stagnation; qi or yin deficiency specifically of the heart; qi or yin or yang deficiency of the kidneys; qi or yin deficiency of the lungs; qi or yin deficiency or fire of the stomach.

Self-diagnosis, unless you are a traditional Chinese medicine practitioner, is never recommended. It takes years of training to be able to understand and properly diagnose these patterns. I would strongly recommend you treat yourself to a consultation with a suitably trained and qualified professional to diagnose your own personal patterns for you, to enable you to tailor your own eating plan accordingly.

However, if this is a step too far for you right now, don't worry, you'll be able to derive lots of benefit from **'the 6 diet'** even if you decide not to incorporate any of the food energetics principles. It's entirely up to you how far you want to tailor your own plan. However, the information in the rest of this section will help you to understand more about how to tailor your own plan if you do decide to get that individualised diagnosis!

Food energetics

The first thing that we should stress about traditional Chinese dietetics or food energetics, is that there are no inherently good or bad foods: there are simply those that are appropriate or inappropriate for each individual. Just as we have already acknowledged that, from a modern nutritional therapy point of view, the balance of carbohydrates to proteins and fats needs to reflect the lifestyle factors for each of us, it is similarly necessary to consider our own needs from a traditional Chinese dietetics perspective.

So, let's look at the actual energetic properties of foods.

Damp foods

We have discussed in some detail now the effects that damp foods can have on our spleen qi, overall health and well-being, body weight, and our appearance.

Of course someone with a perfectly healthy spleen and no weight issues will be able to tolerate some proportion of dampening foods within an overall balanced diet: balanced in terms of qi properties that is! But for anyone needing to lose some weight or body fat, dampening foods are probably the most damaging, both directly damaging to the spleen, and subsequently to the body composition. While it may not be possible to totally eliminate all damp foods at all times, in order to lose weight, and to help heal an impaired spleen, it is essential to keep the use of these foods to an absolute minimum.

This list of foods may contain some surprises, not least because it contains some of the foods that we might normally consider constitute a healthy balanced diet. Initially, the list may seem extremely restrictive, limiting our food choices within the parameters of a normal western diet. However, by experimenting with your diet, you will hopefully come to realise that it is our normal western diet that often limits our food choices. In reality there are many non-dampening foods that we can use. All we have to do is allow ourselves to be more experimental and imaginative in our food selection and cooking. I hope this opens your eyes, as well as hearts and minds to a more wide-ranging and exciting diet than you may have enjoyed so far.

```
DAMP FOODS
  🐾 Wheat and wheat products : including many breads, pastas, pastries, cakes, biscuits (watch
     out for wheat as this is hidden in lots of food products)
  🐾 Dairy products: including milk, yoghurt, cheese, cream, butter, crème fraiche, fromage
     frais.
  🐾 Yeast and yeast products: (again watch out this is hidden in lots of food products, such as
     stock cubes, pates, spreads)
  🐾 Pork and pork products: including ham, bacon, pork sausages
  🐾 Saturated fats
  🐾 Sugar and sweeteners
  🐾 Roasted peanuts
  🐾 Bananas
  🐾 Beer
  🐾 Concentrated juices: especially orange and tomato
     Note: most processed foods, or ready meals are essentially dampening and should be
     avoided
```

Now you've had a chance to cast your eyes over the summary of damp foods listed above, let's discuss each of these foods in turn.

Wheat and Wheat Products

This one is probably the hardest food to imagine being able to remove from a typical Western diet, yet those of us from other cultures should find this little trouble. Many of the staple foods in diets adopted by Western cultures are rich in processed wheat and wheat-based products. Breads, pastries, cakes, biscuits and pastas are all wheat-based products, which must therefore be avoided in order to lose weight. Pasta, I am sure, is a surprise to many, as it is generally considered to be one constituent in a 'healthy balanced diet'. Loved and much used for carbohydrate loading by sportspeople, it is perhaps hard for us to conceive that it is a food best avoided. We probably have less trouble recognising the need to eliminate breads, pastries, cakes and biscuits, as many popular or branded weight-loss diets involve their avoidance too. However, as a refined carbohydrate food, and one increasingly associated with inflammation at that, the avoidance of wheat within **'the 6 diet'** may not feel too prohibitive!

To save the day, there is an increasing range of wheat-free flours available quite readily on our supermarket shelves. Certainly, whole-food shops carry a great range of alternatives for those trying to cater for a wheat-free diet. Corn, maize, tapioca, gram (chickpeas), rice, chestnut, potato, spelt, rye, buckwheat are just a few of the foods that can be milled, and commonly make up wheat-free flours, which may contain one or a combination of these ingredients. Similarly, there is a fascinating, expanding range of wheat-free pastas also available. Pastas made from such ingredients as rice, maize, spelt, buckwheat, corn, and a variety of vegetable starches can easily be found. Again, these may contain one or a combination of ingredients.

In fact, by trying to avoid your usual products, far from finding yourself restricted, you will probably be opening a door to a much more interesting and varied diet than before. Also remember there are other interesting grains such as rice, barley, oatmeal, quinoa, etc. that can be used to add variety to the diet.

Perhaps the most challenging and time-consuming aspect **'the 6 diet'** will be the change in shopping habits. No doubt, as you scour product labels and try to identify appropriate items, you will initially find yourself spending much longer in the supermarket or whole-food shop. This in itself, though, can be a rewarding task, as you will find as you identify new foods previously bypassed and never before considered. After just a few shopping trips, you will be much more adept at spotting appropriate foods, and once again will settle into your new shopping pattern.

Dairy Products

When discussing dairy products with patients in clinic, there always seems to be some confusion about what the term 'dairy' actually means. Simply it is anything made from cows' milk. This includes the milk itself and, yes, even skimmed milk is considered to be dampening. In western research we are now beginning to see links between dairy consumption and inflammation – supporting the traditional Chinese view that it can be harmful in terms of our health.

Whilst it is perfectly likely that most people would understand the dangers of full-fat milk, being used to the incorrect 'low-fat is healthy' mantra, it is probably quite surprising to anyone who regularly uses skimmed milk and skimmed milk products on the understanding that it constitutes the 'healthy option'. Again, **'the 6 diet'** has already debunked the myth of the 'healthy low-fat' option, but there is more to say specifically about skimmed milk products. Here is an excerpt from an article that I have previously written on this very subject:

Research has found that not only will skimmed milk fail to help weight loss but that it might even make you fatter than drinking whole or full-fat milk. As long ago as 2005, researchers reported, 'skim and 1% milk were associated with weight gain, but dairy fat was not'. Two main reasons for this have been put forward: first that fats curb your appetite, and second that they slow down the rate at which sugar is absorbed into your bloodstream, reducing the amount that can be stored as body fat.

If that doesn't make a good enough argument against skimmed milk then consider this: when fat is removed from milk it leaves a bluey-grey colour liquid which is effectively 'painted' to make it white again. This process causes the cholesterol that naturally occurs in milk to become oxidised. Oxidised cholesterol has been linked in in research with a host of disease conditions. Remember what you have already read about oxidative stress?

So both full fat and skimmed milks are, in their respective ways, detrimental to your waistline and your health it seems! It's revealing that modern scientific research supports traditional Chinese dietary advice, which tells us that dairy makes us fat and is bad for health. That's exactly why we should embrace these fabulous ancient principles alongside modern nutritional scientific principles for health and weight loss and give traditional Chinese dietetics its rightful place in modern healthcare.

The same is true of yoghurt. Again, yoghurt is usually considered to be a healthy food, but if made from cows' milk it is still fundamentally a damp food according to traditional Chinese dietetics.

All cheeses made from cows' milk are contraindicated. This includes cottage cheese, which once again is usually considered to be acceptable, and is often advocated by other popular, but flawed, weight-loss plans.

Cream in any form, be it double, single, half, soured, or whipping varieties are dairy products, and as such to be strictly avoided. Other similar products, including crème fraiche and fromage frais fall into the same category, and should also be avoided.

Finally, butter and buttermilk products are contraindicated for anyone avoiding dampening foods. Care should be taken when trying to find substitutes for butter, as many of the spreads available to us often contain some proportion of butter or buttermilk.

However, before you despair, you need to be aware of the alternatives available. Again, there is a wealth of choice when trying to identify acceptable non-dairy products. Remember the term 'dairy' relates to cows. As such goats' milk and milk products are not categorised as 'dairy'. Nor are sheep's or ewes' milk and milk products. Both are considered to be much less dampening than cows' milk products, and as such can be used in moderation. Goats' or ewes' milk, yoghurts and cheeses are increasingly available on supermarket shelves, and many are really delicious!

Alternatively, you may also wish to take a moderate advantage of the growing range of soya products as a substitute for dairy foods. There is a wide selection of soya milks, yoghurts, desserts, creams, cheeses available. Similarly, other plant and cereal-based milk substitutes are increasingly being made, and the range of such is ever growing. These include products made from rice, oats and almonds to name a few of those more commonly available.

Yeast and Yeast-based Products

Possibly, that this is included in the list of damp foods also causes some surprise. However, it really takes only a small leap in imagination to understand the truth of this. Being closely related to moulds, the growth of which we can readily relate to damp conditions, it is easier to think of yeast as a fusty, stagnant, damp substance.

Avoiding yeast is not always as easy as it first appears. Again this relies on some label reading when shopping. Yeast as an ingredient is not merely limited to the obvious foods such as bread. Rather it is contained within many processed food products, including some spreads, pates, and stock-cubes. In order to successfully avoid yeast consumption, it is necessary to become familiar with the list of ingredients contained in a variety of common products.

Pork and Pork Products

This is the only type of meat specifically listed as dampening. However, the Chinese also state that other 'rich' meats are dampening. Unhelpfully, exactly what the term 'rich' meats mean remains unspecified, but it doesn't take a great imagination to picture just what is meant. What I can tell you about this is that a typical rural Chinese diet includes very little red meat, this being limited to just once or twice a week. As such, my advice is to similarly restrict your intake of any red meat, but to more strictly avoid pork.

However, avoiding pork is not always so straight forward. Pork cuts, ham, gammon, and bacon are, of course, all contraindicated. However, sausages, pates, burgers, meat spreads, processed chicken and turkey meats also frequently incorporate some quantity of pork meat or fat. As such, these are also to be avoided. Again, it is most advisable to read labels thoroughly when shopping.

Again, we have evidence that modern western science can support this traditional Chinese viewpoint. Processed meat and meat products, which so often are pork-based (think of packaged ham, pork sausages, bacon etc.) were vilified in our mainstream press early in 2013, having been found in medical research to be a risk factor in the development of serious diseases – many of them which, again, may be associated with inflammation.

Saturated fats

There is probably little surprise that saturated fats are to be avoided on any weight-loss diet. Though, as we have already seen with **'the 6 diet'**, there is a view that saturated fat is not the great villain it has previously been thought. That said, while our bodies can tolerate and deal with some saturated fat, it certainly isn't a recommended food, either for great bodily appearance or performance! It is advisable to limit the consumption of saturated fats for general health and well-being. We are quite familiar with this concept, and probably readily accept the need to avoid saturated fats. However, unlike some other popular weight-loss diets, no restrictions are placed on the consumption of good quality unsaturated fats and oils. It is especially difficult to find a truly unsaturated fat or oil, as probably all contain some saturated proportion. Olive oil is positively encouraged, because as we shall see later, olives are considered to be a beneficial damp-draining food. Other oils, including sesame, pumpkin, sunflower, various nut oils etc. may be used in moderation, as they contain essentially low proportions of saturates – but again, beware too much Omega-6.

This of course is another example of traditional age-old Chinese thinking now resonating closely with the latest in modern nutritional thinking, and another reason why **'the 6 diet'** tells you it is wise to base your own dietary system on a combination of both paradigms!

Sugar and sweeteners

Well, what is there left for us to say about sugar and artificial sweeteners that we haven't already covered in great detail in this book?

Whilst we may not previously have considered sugars to be damp, we are familiar with the need to avoid sugars when attempting to lose weight and improve our health.

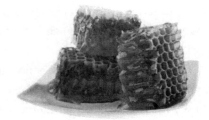

Curiously, the energetic spleen prefers foods having a 'sweet' flavour. However, this concept of 'sweet' describes a natural quality inherent in the food itself. It refers only to foods that are naturally sweet flavoured, and does not at all include foods containing added or processed sweetness, in the form of either natural sugars or artificial sweeteners. In fact, when you have eliminated a large proportion of sugars and sweeteners from your diet, you will begin to recognise the natural sweetness in some unexpected places. For example, it's really amazing how many vegetables actually taste sweet when your taste buds become attuned to natural tastes rather than the intense sweetness of refined sugars and artificial laboratory-made chemical sweeteners. And the more you chew, the more you will release the natural sweet flavours in your foods. You may initially be surprised to learn that a majority of foods are classified as having a sweet flavour within traditional Chinese dietetics, but get into the habit of enjoying natural tastes and you will undoubtedly begin to see why!

Roasted peanuts

Although nuts and seeds are high in calorific value, only roasted peanuts are included in the list of damp foods, and therefore contraindicated. Perhaps this can be explained by the fact that peanuts are not actually nuts — nuts grow in shells on trees, while peanuts grow in pods below ground. More accurately peanuts are classified as a close relation to pulses. The consumption of other nuts, or perhaps I should say real nuts, is not restricted. Indeed, as we shall discover soon, some nuts are thought to be positively beneficial, having damp-draining qualities.

Bananas

The only fruit that appears on the list of damp foods is the banana. As such it is the only fruit that should be avoided, the others eaten in moderation. The reason for this is that bananas are the most starchy of all the fruits, and thus will release a large hit of natural sugars early in the digestive process. Clinical observation confirms that eliminating bananas from the diet is helpful in the treatment of 'damp' conditions.

Beer

The only alcoholic beverage that is considered to be especially dampening is beer. Essentially, this includes all forms of beer: those being lagers, ales, stouts etc. As such, it is the only form of alcoholic drink that is to be strictly avoided. However, whilst wines and spirits may, at least from a traditional Chinese dietetics perspective, be enjoyed in moderation, there is more to say on the subject of them later. As you already know, from **'the 6 diet'** perspective, alcohol in any form, be it beer, wine or spirit, is still a concentrated source of sugar, with the ability to seriously disturb your blood-sugar balance.

Concentrated juices

Perhaps another surprise for most is that concentrated juices are also to be avoided. However, the critical factor here is the massively high levels of fructose that is inherent in any juice, with their concentrated form being especially problematic. Even fresh juices may only be consumed in strict moderation.

Once again, we usually consider juices to be quite healthy compared to other beverages. However, we usually fail to distinguish between concentrated and fresh juices. Often there is little difference between the product packaging used for concentrated and fresh juices. As such, this is yet another occasion when thorough label-reading is an essential factor in shopping.

Damp-resolving foods

Damp-resolving foods, as we have already discussed, are especially useful in helping our bodies to resolve any accumulated internal dampness. Quite how some of these foods work against dampness is difficult to explain. There is little information available in traditional Chinese dietetics texts, probably because this ancient form of medicine, which has evolved over many centuries, developed as a result of close observation of cause and effect.

That said, it is quite obvious from a scientific perspective, how some of the foods help to break down fats. Quite a number of the foods in the list have a sharp or sour taste, and we can easily imagine them to cut through fats or oils deposited within the body tissues. Grapefruit, lemon, onion, radish, turnip, umeboshi plum, and watercress all share this piquant property. Indeed, some weight-loss diets have been built around such foods.

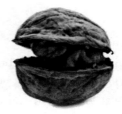

Other foods on the list are known to have diuretic properties, and so are useful to help drain water from the body tissues. Water retention is well known as one cause of bloating, heaviness and oedema. Also, when fatty tissue is waterlogged, we develop the unattractive ripple or orange-peel effect of cellulite. Celery, grapes, lettuce are examples of foods having a gentle diuretic effect on the body.

Once more, I must stress, that while it is useful to incorporate more of these foods into your diet, it is not necessary to limit your diet to include only the foods shown in this list. For example, perhaps you could use pickled lemons as an accompaniment to chicken? Or may be add a teaspoon of umeboshi plum paste to a stir fry?

Replacing normal tea and coffee with one of the teas listed is an especially good start for those who regularly drink warm beverages.

Snacking on the fruits and nuts listed is fine. Or maybe you can be encouraged to be more experimental in cooking, and introduce small changes by adding more of the herbs listed into your favourite recipes?

DAMP-RESOLVING FOODS

- **Vegetables:** beans (especially aduki beans, broad beans, and kidney beans), button mushroom, celery, garlic, lettuce, onion, pumpkin, radish, shitake mushroom, turnip, watercress
- **Fruits:** grape, grapefruit, lemon, olive, pear, umeboshi plum (traditional Japanese pickled plum)
- **Herbs, Spices & Condiments:** fenugreek, garlic, horseradish, liquorice, marjoram, mustard leaf, mustard seed, parsley, peppermint, thyme
- **Grains:** barley, corn, rye
- **Meats and Fish:** anchovy, clam, mackerel, sardine, shrimp
- **Nuts:** almond, walnut
- **Miscellaneous:** buckwheat tea, green tea, jasmine tea, seaweed

Heating foods

As described earlier, the spleen is especially benefited by warming and drier foods. We have already seen how poor spleen qi contributes to our storing excess body fat. Therefore, as well as avoiding damp foods and the excessive use of cold foods, incorporating some damp-draining foods into our diet is also beneficial to ensure the effective and efficient functioning of the spleen. Therefore, to nurture and nourish our spleens we should incorporate drier and gently warming foods into our diets.

However, you should be mindful of the need to avoid an excessive use of these foods if you experience any signs of heat in your body. You definitely need to avoid these foods if you experience the signs or symptoms associated with excess heat in your body, but it is also a consideration in cases where the heat associated with a deficiency of our bodies' cooling mechanisms is experienced. Incorporating more cooling foods, as detailed a little later, may be especially useful where bodily heat is problematic.

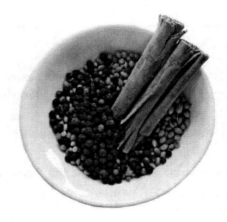

You also need to be aware of these foods in order to maintain a healthy balance day to day between warming and cooling foods in order to meet the respective needs of both your spleen and stomach.

HEATING FOODS

- 🍂 **Vegetables:** caper berries, garlic, kohlrabi, leek, onion, spring onion, squash, sweet potato, sweet rice, turnip
- 🍂 **Fruits:** cherry, lychee, peach
- 🍂 **Herbs, Spices & Condiments:** basil, bay, black pepper, cayenne, chilli pepper, chive seed, coriander seed, dill seed, fennel seed, ginger, mustard leaf, nutmeg, pine kernel, rosemary, spearmint
- 🍂 **Meats and Fish:** anchovy, chicken, lamb, lamb kidney, mussel, mutton, shrimp, trout
- 🍂 **Nuts:** chestnut, walnut
- 🍂 **Miscellaneous:** amasake, coconut milk, soya oil, vinegar, wines, spirits

Yin-tonifying foods

These are the foods that can help to strengthen our innate cooling mechanisms – i.e. our Yin qi. As our Yin qi is tonified and our bodies' abilities to maintain an appropriate cooling mechanism improve, the heat arising from the deficiency will naturally diminish. Until this is re-established it may be useful to also avoid excessively heating foods as listed above, and incorporate more cooling foods as listed a little later.

YIN-TONIFYING FOODS

- 🍂 **Vegetables:** asparagus, kidney bean, pea, string bean, tomato
- 🍂 **Fruits:** apple, lemon, mango, pear, pineapple, pomegranate
- 🍂 **Meats and Fish:** crab, duck, rabbit
- 🍂 **Miscellaneous:** chicken egg, duck egg, tofu

Cooling foods

As discussed earlier, an excessive consumption of energetically cold foods will, eventually, deplete the spleen qi. Therefore, it is important to know which foods are considered to be cooling, in order to ensure their appropriate and moderate use. It is by no means essential to pay as much attention to these foods as to damp foods. It is, however, necessary to consider these foods in order to tailor your diet to your own unique needs. Therefore, I cannot stress enough at this point that it is an excessive use of these foods that should be avoided.

Remember though, in addition, that an excessive use of raw foods – as these are also essentially cooling – is also to be avoided.

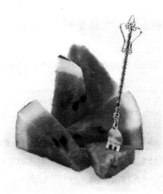

All foods, if eaten raw, fall into this category. Again I stress the word excessive here. Any moderate use of cold or raw foods should be fine, except where signs of cold exist in your body. This cold may be associated with an excess of internal cold, or as a result of your innate warming mechanism – your Yang-qi – being impaired.

In either case, you may choose to incorporate more warming or heating foods until your Yang-qi is sufficiently restored and your own internal warming mechanism re-established.

COOLING FOODS

- 🍂 **Vegetables:** asparagus, aubergine, bamboo shoots, lettuce, kidney beans, mung beans, mung beansprouts, pea, potato, string bean, tomato, yam
- 🍂 **Fruits:** apple, grapefruit, lemon, mango, melon, pear, pineapple, pomegranate, watermelon
- 🍂 **Herbs, Spices & Condiments:** elderflower, peppermint, salt
- 🍂 **Grains:** millet
- 🍂 **Meats and Fish:** clam, crab, cuttlefish, duck, oyster
- 🍂 **Miscellaneous:** chicken eggs, duck eggs, tofu

*Note: if you read similar lists in other books about traditional Chinese dietetics, it is likely you will find other foods classified as cold or cooling. However, some are also dampening, and so, for **'the 6 diet'** purposes, I have omitted them from this list.*

Yang-tonifying foods

These are the foods that can help to strengthen our innate warming mechanisms – i.e. our Yang qi. As our Yang qi is tonified and our bodies' abilities to maintain an appropriate warming mechanism improve, the cold arising from the deficiency will naturally diminish. Until this is re-established it may be useful to also avoid excessively cooling foods as listed above, and incorporate more warming or heating foods as listed earlier.

YANG-TONIFYING FOODS

- **Vegetables:** garlic, savory
- **Herbs, Spices & Condiments:** aniseed, basil, cardamom, chive seed, cinnamon, clove, dill seed, fennel seed, fenugreek seed, ginger, nutmeg, rosemary, sage, star anise, thyme
- **Grains:** quinoa
- **Meats and Fish:** anchovy, goat, kidney, lamb, lobster, mutton, shrimp, trout, venison
- **Nuts:** chestnut, pistachio, walnut

Qi-forming foods

Where a need to tonify or strengthen qi is indicated the following foods should be incorporated into your diet. As with all the lists provided in respect of traditional Chinese dietetics, it is important to understand that emphasising these foods does not limit you to only these foods – rather incorporating them where you can is especially useful, and making sure you consume something from the lists at least once each day is appropriate.

QI-FORMING FOODS

- **Vegetables:** carrot, chickpea, lentil, potato, sweet potato, shiitake mushroom, squash, yam
- **Fruits:** cherry, date, fig, grape, longan
- **Herbs, Spices & Condiments:** liquorice, sage
- **Grains:** millet, oats, quinoa, rice
- **Meats and Fish:** beef, chicken, eel, goose, herring, mackerel, octopus, pheasant, pigeon, rabbit, sardine, sturgeon, trout, venison
- **Nuts:** almond, coconut
- **Miscellaneous:** chicken egg, ginseng, microalgae, milk, molasses, pigeon egg, royal jelly, tempeh, tofu

Blood-forming foods

Where a need to tonify or strengthen blood is indicated the following foods should be incorporated into your diet.

BLOOD-FORMING FOODS
- **Vegetables:** aduki bean, beetroot, dark leafy greens, kidney bean, spinach, watercress
- **Fruits:** apricot, date, fig, grape
- **Herbs, Spices & Condiments:** nettle, parsley
- **Meats and Fish:** beef, chicken, liver, oyster, sardine
- **Miscellaneous:** chicken egg

Qi-moving foods

Where signs and symptoms indicating qi stagnation exist, the following foods can usefully be incorporated to promote qi circulation, and re-establish a smooth flow of qi around your body. As you will note, almost all are herbs, spices or condiments, which makes it really easy to begin to incorporate them more into your cooking. The additional flavours that you can bring to your meals very easily should be motivation enough to experiment with this particular list of ingredients.

QI-MOVING FOODS
- **Vegetables:** carrot, radish
- **Herbs, Spices & Condiments:** basil, caraway, cardamom, cayenne, chive, clove, coriander, dill seed, garlic, marjoram, mustard leaf, star anise, turmeric
- **Miscellaneous:** orange peel, tangerine peel

Blood-moving foods

Where signs and symptoms indicating blood stasis exist, the following foods can usefully be incorporated to promote blood circulation around your body.

BLOOD-MOVING FOODS

- **Vegetables:** aubergine, kohlrabi, leek, onion, radish, scallion, turnip
- **Fruits:** peach
- **Herbs, Spices & Condiments:** chilli pepper, chive, hawthorn berry, mustard leaf, saffron, turmeric, vinegar
- **Grain:** sweet rice
- **Meats and Fish:** crab, shark, sturgeon
- **Nuts:** chestnut
- **Miscellaneous:** amasake, brown sugar, butter, chicken egg, rose

---

Balancing the needs of your stomach and spleen

The need for balance

We have now looked in detail at the functions, the likes and the dislikes of both our stomachs and spleens, and the foods that we can use to benefit our bodily appearance and health. So it is clear that in order for our bodies to be able to process food properly, enabling us to appropriately manage our weight and health, we must equally meet the needs of both these organs. The relationship between the two is essentially symbiotic, the qi of the spleen and stomach is really the same energy source and thus the organs are mutually dependant such that when one is impaired the other will quickly become so.

When a traditional Chinese medicine practitioner designs a treatment for any condition one of the considerations will be to balance the patient's qi. Similarly, when designing your diet, you also need to consider the issue of balance. Where your spleen and stomach are already in balance, the main aim is to maintain that balance. Where an imbalance exists, the main aim is to adjust the diet to satisfy both your spleen and stomach, but paying more attention to one or the other where an imbalance is evident.

Many lifestyle issues may affect the balance of our qi, and consequently the balance of health between the spleen and stomach organs and their respective qi. Studying, stress, worry, the pace of life, natural aging, overwork are but a few of the causes ensuring that you need to keep a constant watch on your own energetic state – especially when trying to lose weight or improve health. One really important thing to note is that medicines also have energetic properties. Because these are often administered orally – taken in liquid, tablet or capsule form – they are easily able to disturb the digestive processes by affecting the qi of the spleen and stomach in the same way as foods. Antibiotics especially are energetically cold and dampening. This means that if you catch an infection and take antibiotic medicines you are introducing external dampness into your body. Many other drugs are energetically hot, and therefore provide a source of external heat affecting your stomach when taken orally.

Because your qi is in a constant state of flux it is necessary to pay regular attention to your qi needs, and to those of your spleen and stomach. What you require today may be different tomorrow. This makes perfect sense: we have already discussed the different day to day needs in respect of carbohydrates, proteins and other nutrients depending upon your different daily activities, and balancing your qi is just the same!

Achieving balance

In analysing the various likes and dislikes of both organs, we can recognise that there is some common ground between our spleen and stomach. For example, both organs are benefited by a regular and relaxed eating pattern. Both are equally injured by over-thinking or mental exertion. Therefore, by ensuring our eating environment is suitable, and by relaxing our minds we can easily and equally benefit both our spleens and stomachs.

However, we can also see, by comparing the likes and dislikes of the two organs, that some of them seem to be in conflict. Our spleens prefer warm, dry foods, and our stomachs prefer cooling, moist foods. Excess fluids can injure our spleens' qi, but fluids are essential to support the qi functions of our stomachs. This is where we have to work carefully to strike a balance, recognising the need to adopt moderation in our dietary habits in order to benefit both organs, or at least to injure neither! Essentially, foods should neither be extremely heating or cooling, unless respective signs of cold or heat arise, in which case heating or cooling foods can be used therapeutically to resolve problems. We should take in only small amounts of fluids when eating so as not to upset our spleens, but ensure we drink plenty of fluids between meals to support our stomach fluids.

Of course, in achieving balance between the two organs, it is useful to be able to recognise when they are not in balance so that appropriate adjustments can be made. When embarking on this process it is best to expect that imbalance may at some time occur. After all, if qi is never static then it is probably unrealistic to expect that there is no need to adjust our diets from time to time in order to maintain balance between our spleens and stomachs.

It is not uncommon for individuals to find that when they avoid the use of damp foods, and thereby begin to reduce the amount of internal damp accumulated in the body, signs of heat will begin to surface. This is because dampness is good at keeping a lid on heat and fire. Rather like a chip-pan fire – all it takes is a damp cloth to contain the fire. However, if you remove the cloth before the fire has properly died out, the flames will spontaneously flare again, and the signs of that contained heat will be immediately apparent. In just the same way, if you remove excess dampness by gently warming and nourishing the spleen, it is quite possible to reveal stomach heat. It is likely that the heat has been there all along, but simply masked by the dampness. It is possible to inadvertently over-warm your digestive system. By paying proper attention to warming your spleen qi, you can unwittingly neglect your stomach qi, giving rise to the warning signs of heat.

Signs that your stomach energy is becoming too hot may include the following:

- discomfort, fullness, or pain in the epigastrium, especially after food
- feeling of heat in the epigastrium, especially after food
- hiccupping or belching
- indigestion, acid reflux, or heartburn
- regurgitation of food, nausea and vomiting
- constipation or hot diarrhoea
- infrequent or scant urination, with concentrated or dark yellow coloured urine
- headaches associated with food, or after eating
- sour / rotten taste – where this is definitely not associated with dental problems
- bad breath / halitosis – where this is definitely not associated with dental problems
- sore or bleeding gums – where this is definitely not associated with dental problems
- toothache – where this is not simply associated with tooth decay

Not everyone having stomach heat or fire will experience all of these signs or symptoms. Nor do many of these signs and symptoms always indicate the presence of stomach heat or fire. As noted above, some may in fact be as a result of poor dental health or oral hygiene. Headaches may stem from many causes. However, if some of these signs and symptoms begin to show up after reducing the damp content of your diet, it is a possible indication of stomach heat.

In order to counteract this, you should gently cool your diet by incorporating some of the cooling foods previously listed. Of course, if you over-cool the diet, paying too much attention to tackling stomach heat, it is also possible then to tip the balance the other way. Remember, an unhealthy spleen can generate internal dampness where its transformation function fails. You do not need to actually consume energetically damp foods or substances to accumulate internal dampness.

We have already discussed the signs and symptoms of internal dampness accumulation – so please be vigilant.

Also, by over-cooling your stomach, it is possible to create a condition of stomach cold. This is usually as a result of over-consumption of extremely cold or chilled foods and drink, and as we have already said, may cause acute or chronic signs and symptoms.

The signs and symptoms most commonly associated with this include:

- discomfort, fullness, or pain in the epigastrium, especially after food
- sensation of cold in the epigastrium, especially after food
- midriff cold to touch
- nausea either while eating or soon after food
- belching or indigestion during or soon after food
- acute attack of vomiting soon after eating
- watery diarrhoea with undigested food present in stools

Most of the time you will be able to ensure balance by consuming a wide range of foods in moderation – neither veering too much towards excessively heating or cooling foods, and maintaining an energetic neutrality in your diet.

I cannot stress enough though that proper diagnosis in the traditional Chinese medicine sense is a complex matter, and not really for the lay person. **'the 6 diet'** provides you with resources to achieve a dietary plan satisfying both the modern nutritional therapy and traditional Chinese dietetics requirements especially for you. It takes full account of your own individual and unique needs from both perspectives.

Alternately you may seek professional input from both a nutritional therapist and practitioner of traditional Chinese dietetics to help you to make proper sense of your needs and solutions.

Chapter 4:

Creating your unique food plan

Overview of the steps to create your plan

This section of **'the 6 diet'** is REALLY exciting, because here you can turn all that new knowledge and thinking about food into action: action specifically for YOU!

It takes about 12 weeks to make a real change in terms of body composition. So the first thing to bear in mind is that it will take just 12 weeks of serious committed effort to achieve fabulous, lasting, beneficial results! That's right – in just 12 weeks' time you will be a whole different you! And you'll begin to see benefits almost immediately – after just a few days you'll probably begin to see signs of positive change that will show you the power of **'the 6 diet'**!

There are a few stages to getting going, and we'll look at all of them in turn so that by the end of this section your plan is complete:

- Setting your goals
- Calculating how much food you need
- Establishing which foods you need
- Fine tuning your plan
- Portion selections
- Working out when you need to eat

In this chapter we'll explore in detail exactly HOW to work out everything you need to create your plan. To get this right you will have to spend a little time and effort, but the more precisely you can define your plan the greater your success will be. Remember – the key to success is having a plan tailored for you, so don't be tempted to copy what anyone else does with their plan!

So let's get to your goal setting!

Setting your goals

Knowing what you want to achieve is crucial to your ability to achieve it!

Having vague notions of 'losing weight', 'being more healthy', 'having more vitality' or even 'lowering my blood sugar' are not motivational. They really don't give you much to aim for. What's more, how will you ever know when you've succeeded?

So, be clear! You wouldn't be reading this if you didn't want to improve your body in some way – be it in relation to your appearance, health, performance, fitness etc. Spending a little time defining specifically what it is that you don't like now and what it is that you want to be different in the near future will give you a clarity that enables you to know exactly where you are in relation to your targets. Seeing yourself making positive headway towards your ideal body will spur you on along the way – and ultimately tell you when it's time to really celebrate the new you!

On the next page is your goal chart. Using this format will help you to capture your goals / targets, and chart your progress on your 12 week journey! Of course – depending on your individual goals and your baseline now – you might not achieve everything you want to in 12 weeks, but that's OK.

After 12 weeks you'll need to reassess your baseline, because you'll have made such positive inroads towards your goals that your original starting point is no longer valid. As your body changes it needs your plan to change too! **'the 6 diet'** has a great ability to adapt as you change, which means it's truly your plan for life! There is no wondering what to do when you've reached your goals, because **'the 6 diet'** has the answer: there is always a new goal – and one day soon it will be to simply maintain the fabulous new you!

Goals and Progress Tracker

Name: *A.N. Example* **Date:** *Today!*

Baseline Measures	Weight: 10 stones 10lbs	Fat Mass: BMI 29	Symptoms: *Mid-afternoon energy dip* *Waking at 3:00am* *Blood glucose 52*
Goals / Targets	Weight: 9 stones 4lbs	Fat Mass: BMI 25	Symptoms: *Sustained energy* *Not waking in the night* *Blood glucose 40*
WEEK 1	*10 stones 8lbs*	*BMI 28*	*Detox headache?*
WEEK 2	*10 stones 7lbs*	*BMI 28*	*Energy lasting until 10pm*
WEEK 3	*10 stones 5lbs*	*BMI 28*	*Sleeping more deeply*
WEEK 4	*10 stones 3lbs*	*BMI 27*	*Sleeping through all night*

Your baseline measures

In Chapter 2 we looked in detail at body composition. Knowing your own body composition is one of the best ways of establishing your own baseline measures – and ultimately once you know them, your ideal body composition helps you to establish specific targets and goals. **'the 6 diet'**, therefore, encourages you to assess and understand your own body composition.

If you have the resources in your locality then I would encourage you to get as comprehensive a check as you can find and afford. But at the very least you can work out your own BMI, by measuring your height and current weight and performing the calculation using the formula that I have shown in Chapter 2. You can also very simply calculate your hip to waist ratio also as shown in Chapter 2. Both the BMI and hip:waist ratio measures will give you a rudimentary measure of where you are, and by comparing yourself with the healthy ranges that I have shown you, set yourself some reasonable goals.

Your goals

Remember – a healthy loss of body fat can only happen at a steady 1-2lbs per. week. Beyond that you will be very likely burning your lean tissues instead of body fat. So if weight loss is indeed one of your targets ensure your goal is a healthy one!

Of course – your target doesn't have to include weight loss at all, and it may even include some weight gain! It may involve a conversion of existing fat mass to lean tissue mass rather than a change in overall weight, or it may focus on other health or vitality indicators of your own choosing. You will find **'the 6 diet'** will help you to achieve better blood sugar control, more energy and vitality and better health even if your weight is already optimum!

It's entirely up to you! **'the 6 diet'** will help you to deliver a wide range of possible improvements as you will no doubt have learned from your reading so far in this book.

How much food do you need?

This really depends on how much energy your body needs! Energy that is in the ordinary sense, not the qi sense.

Again, we have already talked about how your own body composition influences this, so the more accurately you can know your body composition the more precisely you can calculate your energetic needs.

The starting point for calculating your own energy needs is to work out your BMR. Just to remind you – this is the amount of energy your body needs simply to keep you alive: your Basal Metabolic Rate. Once you know your BMR, factoring in your daily activity levels, and the energy requirements to serve them, helps you to calculate your overall needs, i.e. your overall Metabolic Rate.

Calculating your BMR

There are several ways to calculate your BMR. Some of the methods we discussed for assessing your body composition will calculate your BMR for you, precisely based on your own ratios of fat mass and lean mass. However, if you are unable to benefit from those methods, then there are some formula-based methods that you can use, based on knowing some much more easily obtainable measures. A reasonably accurate method of manually calculating your BMR is the Harris-Benedict formula.

The Harris Benedict equation is a calorie formula using the factors of height, weight, age, and sex to determine BMR. This makes it more accurate than determining calorie needs based on total bodyweight alone, but it cannot take into account your individual percentages of lean mass and fat mass. Therefore, this equation will be very accurate in many cases, but is not completely adequate for those with extremely muscular physiques, as it will underestimate your energy needs, or for those with who are carrying extreme amounts of body fat, as it will overestimate your energy needs. If you think you fall into one of these extreme categories then a more comprehensive assessment of your body composition is called for.

For most though, this formula will be accurate enough to enable you to get those great results that you desire!

So you will need to determine your:

- Height (Ht)
- Weight (Wt)
- Age
- Sex i.e. male (M) or female (F)

Then run your results through one of these formulae:

Females:
Using Metric measures – i.e. height in centimetres (cm) and weight in kilograms (kg)
BMR = 655 + (9.6 x wt in kg) + (1.8 x ht in cm) - (4.7 x age in years)

Using Imperial measures – i.e. height in inches (ins) and weight in pounds (lbs)
BMR = 655 + (4.35 x weight in lbs) + (4.7 x height in ins) - (4.7 x age in years)

Males:
Using Metric measures – i.e. height in centimetres (cm) and weight in kilograms (kg)
BMR = 66 + (13.7 x wt in kg) + (5 x ht in cm) - (6.8 x age in years)

Using Imperial measures – i.e. height in inches (ins) and weight in pounds (lbs)
BMR = 66 + (6.23 x weight in lbs) + (12.7 x height in ins) - (6.8 x age in years)

Here are a few of examples:

Female, aged 51 years, weight 10 stones 10lbs (150lbs), height 5 feet 1 inch (61 ins):
BMR = 655 + (4.35 x 150) + (4.7 x 61) - (4.7 x 51) =

    655 + (652.5)   + (286.7)   - (239.7)   =   1354.5 calories energy

Female, aged 51 years, weight 68 kilograms (kg), height 155 centimetres (cms) :
BMR = 655 + (9.6 x 68) + (1.8 x 155) - (4.7 x 51) =

    655 + (652.8)   + (279)   - (239.7)   =   1347.1 calories energy

These calculations show that whether you use metric or imperial measurements, the formulae will be accurate to within a few calories – an insignificant amount in **'the 6 diet'** terms.

And examples for the men:

Male, aged 53 years, weight 12 stones 4lbs (172lbs), height 6 feet 1 inch (73 ins):
BMR = 66 + (6.23 x 172) + (12.7 x 73) - (6.8 x 53) =

    66 + (1071.56)   + (927.1)   - (360.4)   =   1704.26 calories energy

Male, aged 53 years, weight 78 kilograms (kg), height 185 centimetres (cm):
BMR = 66 + (13.7 x 78) + (5 x 185) - (6.8 x 53) =

    66 + (1068.6)   + (925)   - (360.4)   =   1699.2 calories energy

Again, this shows that both imperial and metric measures will give equally significant results.

If you have had your body composition more thoroughly measured and you know your lean body mass, then you can more accurately calculate your BMR manually too. The formula from Katch & McArdle takes into account lean mass and therefore is more accurate than a formula based on total body weight. The Harris Benedict equation has separate formulas for men and women because men generally have a higher level of lean body mass and this is factored into the men's formula. Since the Katch & McArdle formula specifically takes into account the lean body mass then the same formula applies equally to both men and women. Remember, we said previously that only lean body mass burns energy – fat mass is essentially a store of energy! So this formula is much simpler, as long as you know the amount of lean mass you have in terms of weight in kilograms:

BMR (men and women) = 370 + (21.6 X lean mass in kg)

So for example:
Female, weight 120 lbs. (54.5 kilos), body fat percentage is 20% (24 lbs. fat, 96 lbs. lean), lean mass is 96 lbs. (43.6 kilos)

BMR = 370 + (21.6 X 43.6) = 1312 calories

Factoring in your activity levels

Once you have determined your BMR you will need to assess just how physically active you are on average on a daily basis.

The amount of activity you undertake will massively change the amount of energy your body needs to maintain itself just the way it is.

The Harris-Benedict formula helps with this too, and the same activity multipliers can be used on the BMR regardless of the method used to calculate it initially.

To determine your own multiplier, you need to be honest about the type of daily activity profile that fits you. Choose from the following list developed by Harris-Benedict:

- Sedentary = little or no exercise, desk job
- Lightly active = light exercise/sports 1-3 days per. wk
- Moderately active = moderate exercise/sports 3-5 days per. wk
- Very active = hard exercise/sports 6-7 days per. wk
- Extremely active = hard daily exercise/sports & physical job or 2 x day training, i.e marathon, contest etc.

Once you have determined which you are, then use the appropriate multiplier to determine your own actual overall metabolic rate:

Sedentary = BMR X 1.2
Lightly active = BMR X 1.375
Moderately active = BMR X 1.55

Very active = BMR X 1.725

Extremely active = BMR X 1.9

Taking our female example from before, say she has a desk job, but goes to the gym once each week, and walks her dog for 20 minutes each day. It would probably be fair to classify her as being lightly active.

So we would multiply her BMR of say 1350 calories by 1.375 to give an overall metabolic rate of 1856.25 calories of energy.

This means that simply in order to fuel her body, to meet its needs to stay exactly the same weight as now, she needs to consume about 1850 calories every day. Of course, if there are days when she decides to take more exercise, then on those days only she will be able to take more calories, and if she rests all day she needs less. The multipliers show just how much more or less are required for different levels of activity of course.

Adjusting energy consumption to meet your weight goals

Once you know your own overall metabolic rate, then you need to think about your own targets again.

If you want to remain at the same weight, then you already know how much you need to each in terms of energy.

If however your goals include some weight loss, then you will need to consume fewer calories than your body needs, so that it can begin the process of satisfying the shortfall by releasing energy from your own body fat stores. *Crucially, to ensure you only burn your fat mass, and leave your lean mass as intact as possible, you will have to be very clever about just how much less energy you take in the form of food.* Reducing your calorific intake by too much means that you will lose weight too quickly – meaning that you will be adversely affecting your body composition. Remember the golden rule that ensuring you only lose between 1-2lbs weight per. week helps to protect your body composition. So your aim should be to reduce your calorific intake only to this extent.

Typically starting by reducing your daily calorific intake to be about 500 calories per. day less than your own overall metabolic rate is a great starting point. So, simply subtract 500 from your activity adjusted score! However, if you find that you begin to lose weight too quickly then adjust this upwards again in small increments, of say 100 calories, until you reach your own optimum amount, ensuring this beneficial rate of weight loss.

A possibly surprising fact about starvation or serious abrupt calorie-reduction is that it can dramatically reduce BMR by up to 30 per cent. So those restrictive low-calorie weight loss diets, operating on some of the fundamentally flawed bases that **'the 6 diet'** has already alerted you to, may cause your BMR to drop by as much as 20%. This means that it becomes harder to lose weight as you progress with the diet, and because your body is unable to use so many calories, you really have to eat less just to maintain your weight loss. Even then, although you eat less your body still tends to store fat. You can also easily see from this why some diets are potentially so damaging to your body composition. It is quite common for those who embark on slimming diets to limit their energy intake to 1000 or even less. Shockingly, some of those branded diets that require you to only consume their own proprietary shakes, bars, soups etc. limit your daily calorific intake to somewhere between 500 and 800 calories. Of course they result in high levels of weight loss quickly! *Of course they are absolutely unhealthy, and have the potential to seriously affect your BMR and body composition, leading to all the health issues that we have already discussed – and now you can clearly see why!*

By considering your body composition in the way that we do, and ensuring your journey improves your body composition, the new, leaner, more muscular you will actually have a higher BMR, and require more calories, rather than less, to maintain your new body.

If your goals include some weight gain, then of course you will need to eat more energy than your body needs. Again, start with consuming about 500 calories per. day *more* than your own overall metabolic rate to ensure a healthy rate of weight gain, and adjust it accordingly.

Some other factors

Several factors may temporarily affect your body's energetic needs, because they can temporarily alter your BMR.

Body Temperature

For every increase of 0.5°C in internal temperature of the body, the BMR increases by about 7 per cent. The chemical reactions in the body actually occur more quickly at higher temperatures. So a patient with a fever of 42°C (about 4°C above normal) would have an increase of about 50 per cent in BMR. Having an illness, even such as a cold or flu, where your temperature is elevated will cause you to temporarily burn more calories.

External temperature

Temperature outside the body also affects the BMR. Exposure to cold temperature causes an increase in the BMR, so as to create the extra heat needed to maintain the body's internal temperature. A short exposure to hot temperature has little effect on the body's metabolism as it is compensated mainly by increased heat loss. But prolonged exposure to heat can raise BMR, in the same way as when we experience a febrile illness as shown in the preceding paragraph.

Exercise

Physical exercise not only influences body weight by burning calories, it also helps raise your BMR by building extra lean tissue, and improving your body composition. Lean tissue is more metabolically demanding than fat tissue – remember lean mass uses energy whereas fat mass doesn't. With a more muscular body composition you burn more calories even when sleeping. We will explain later why exercise is a crucial part of **'the 6 diet'**.

Which foods should you eat?

Now understand why eating for optimum health and weight loss means so much more than simply counting calories. *What* those calories are made up of is crucial to ensure we improve and maintain a great body composition, optimum health and well-being. We've already looked at all the reasons why, from both a modern western nutritional perspective, and incorporating the valuable wisdom inherent in traditional Chinese dietetics. So, for sure, we need to think about the *amount* of food we consume in energetic terms, but now let's take a look at how we can really optimise our dietary plan for the very best results in terms of body composition, health and well-being.

A varied diet is key

It only takes a cursory glance at the information provided in Chapter 3 to realise that a varied diet really is key to ensuring a proper cross section of nutrients is consumed. In order to achieve a full complement of amino acids to ensure your complete protein intake, a modest amount of animal-based protein is required OR a combination of plant-based protein-rich foods OR, of course, a combination of animal and plant-based foods. Similarly, in order to benefit from all the vitamins, minerals and antioxidants that your body needs for optimum health, a wide range of fruits, vegetables, nuts and seeds, wholegrains and pulses need to be incorporated into your food plan. The ratios of different foods are also important – ensuring that to benefit your body composition and overall health and well-being you adopt an approach of consuming low levels of high GI carbohydrates, lots of proteins and adequate fats and slow-release complex carbohydrates.

If that sounds complicated, well **'the 6 diet'** makes it very easy.

By grouping foods into categories for you, all you need to do is to ensure you select a pre-determined number of portions from each on a daily basis according to your planned activities for the day.

The categories are:

- Animal-based complete proteins (or vegetarian substitutes)
- Dairy (which I have separated out from other animal-based protein foods for reasons I will come on to explain)
- Wholegrains
- Pulses
- Non-starchy vegetables
- Starchy vegetables
- Fruit
- Nuts and seeds
- Healthy fats

The number of portions that you require from each category depends upon the overall energy intake you have calculated for yourself and the types of activities you will perform that day, and again **'the 6 diet'** has devised the guidelines to make it easy for you.

I have already taken the liberty of building in some of the traditional Chinese dietetics principles along the way – so if some food categories look incomplete then this is the likely reason. For example, you won't find pork or pork-based products listed with other meats: as the most dampening meat it is inappropriate for anyone committed to health and weight-loss. However, if you are convinced that you have no signs of internal dampness, from a traditional Chinese medicine perspective, and weight loss is not one of your goals, then you may of course incorporate pork, in appropriate portion sizes if desired.

Let's take a look at each category in turn:

Animal-based complete proteins (or vegetarian substitutes)

We have looked in close detail at the reasons why your body needs a complete complement of amino acids on a daily basis. Your body cannot store amino acids, yet it uses them every day to support many bodily functions. With few exceptions, plant-based protein-rich foods are not complete proteins – they do not contain all the essential amino acids.

The foods in this category will deliver all the essential amino acids you need, so ensuring you take appropriate portions from this category gives you peace of mind that you have that base covered. However, red meat remains controversial due to its high saturated fat content. The results of a study by Harvard University, published in 2012, suggest that red meat should be eaten only occasionally – say 10% of the time. This again fits in well with the traditional Chinese dietetics understanding of all 'rich' meats being essentially dampening, and therefore red meat should be kept to minimum levels as part of a weight-loss orientated plan.

Complete Proteins
A typical portion should deliver about 150 calories of energy.
If oil or fats are used in cooking, these must be taken as part of the fat allowance for the day.

Food item	Amount in a single portion
Eggs	2 whole large size – yolk and whites
Oily fish, e.g. mackerel, herring, sardine,	Mackerel 80 grams raw weight Others 100 grams raw weight
Pink fish, e.g. salmon, tuna, trout	100 grams raw weight
White fish, e.g. cod, haddock, skate, plaice, halibut, sea bass	160-180 grams raw weight
Shellfish	180 grams raw weight
Poultry: [1] 🦀 Chicken breast, no skin 🦀 Turkey, no skin 🦀 Duck, no skin 🦀 Goose, no skin	Chicken / turkey 130 grams raw weight Duck 120 grams raw weight Goose 90 grams raw weight

Lamb, lean*² (i.e. fat trimmed to no more than 1-2mm)	80 grams raw weight
Beef, very lean *²	100 grams raw weight
Venison	130 grams raw weight
Rabbit	130 grams raw weight
Tofu	200 grams raw soft 150 grams raw firm For branded tofu products refer to package labelling to determine appropriate quantity
Soya or other similar vegetarian burger / sausage	For branded products refer to package labelling to determine appropriate quantity
Textured Vegetable Protein (TVP)	For branded products refer to package labelling to determine appropriate quantity
Tempeh	80 grams raw weight
Amaranth *³	40 grams raw weight
Quinoa *³	40 grams raw weight

Notes: *¹ *Skin contains high levels of saturated fats, and should be discarded before cooking*

*² *Due to its high levels of saturated fats, only extremely lean red meats such as lamb or beef should be consumed no more than once per. week*

*³ *Included here as well as in grains, in recognition that they provide complete proteins and are therefore valuable vegetarian sources*

Dairy

This is an interesting category – because, as we have seen, all dairy products are considered to be dampening from a traditional Chinese dietetics perspective, and in a western scientific sense are have been associated with inflammatory disease. For most people with either a health or weight loss goal dairy products are therefore probably inappropriate.

There are some reasonable dairy substitutes available on the market, but a word of caution is required: some soya and non-soya products are high in sugars. Especial care is needed when selecting such products. Both dairy and dairy-substitute products are included in this category to provide scope for those who need to avoid the dampening qi qualities of cows' milk produce. In this table I have only included full-fat cows' milk, taking into account our earlier discussion of the potential dangers of skimmed milk products.

Dairy A typical portion should deliver about 80-90 calories of energy. Low-fat products should absolutely be avoided for all your familiar **'the 6 diet'** purposes!	
Food item	**Amount in a single portion**
Cows' milk	Whole milk 150 grams (5 fl oz)
Goats' milk	120 grams (4 fl oz)
Sheep's milk	80 grams (2.5 fl oz)
Unsweetened soya milk	Approximately 180 grams For branded products refer to package labelling to determine appropriate quantity
Plain yoghurt from whole cows' milk *[4]	150 grams
Plain yoghurt from goats' milk	120 grams
Plain yoghurt from sheep's milk	80 grams
Unsweetened soya yoghurt substitute	For branded products refer to package labelling to determine appropriate quantity
Cheese from cows' milk: *[5]	Hard: 20 grams Soft: 25 grams
Cheeses from goats' milk: *[5]	Hard: 20 grams Soft: 30 grams
Cheeses from sheep's milk: *[5]	Hard: 20 grams Soft: 20 grams
Feta Cheese	30 grams
Mozzarella	25 grams
Ricotta	40 grams

Notes: *[4] This is yoghurt from whole milk, and does not include low-fat or fat-free products, as these will likely contain too much sugar or other inappropriate carbohydrates

*[5] As there are many varieties of cheeses, these figures represent average values

Wholegrains

Refined grains are to be completely avoided due to their damaging effects on blood-sugar balance, therefore only whole-grains are to be included in strict moderation within your eating plan.

Also remember that wheat and wheat products are being increasingly linked with inflammatory disease, and are considered to be dampening according to traditional Chinese dietetics. For most people with a health or weight loss goal these are therefore probably inappropriate. They are included here though, for those who have no such restriction of wheat consumption.

Wholegrains	
A typical portion should deliver about 100 calories of energy.	
Flours, meals, pastas etc. all relate to uncooked weight. If oil or fats are used in cooking, these must be taken as part of the fat allowance for the day.	
Food item	**Amount in a single portion**
Whole wheat	
Flour	30 grams
Bread	1 slice
Pitta / tortilla wrap	Half
Pasta	25 grams
Spelt	
Flour	30 grams
Bread	1 slice
Pasta	25 grams
Rye	
Flour	30 grams
Crackers	3 crackers
Bread	1 slice
Oats	
Porridge oats	30 grams
Oatmeal	30 grams
Oatcakes	2 oatcakes
Barley	

🌰 Pearl	30 grams	
🌰 Meal	30 grams	
Buckwheat		
🌰 Flour	30 grams	
🌰 Groats	30 grams	
🌰 Pasta	25 grams	
Millet	25 grams	
Rice		
🌰 Brown	25 grams	
🌰 Basmati	25 grams	
🌰 Wild	25 grams	
Amaranth	25 grams	
Quinoa	30 grams	
Bulgar wheat	30 grams	
Maize meal	30 grams	

Pulses

Pulses	
A typical portion should deliver about 100 calories of energy.	
All values represent raw weight, unless otherwise specified.	
If oil or fats are used in cooking, these must be taken as part of the fat allowance for the day.	

Food item	Amount in a single portion
Lentils	30 grams
Peas	
Split	30 grams
Green	120 grams
Chickpeas	
Whole	30 grams
Hummus	60 grams (approx 4 tablespoons)
Kidney beans	30 grams
Broad beans	30 grams
Pinto beans	30 grams
Aduki beans	30 grams
Cannellini beans	30 grams
Black beans	30 grams
Haricot beans	30 grams
Mung beans	30 grams
Butter beans	30 grams

Non-starchy Vegetables

A wide selection of vegetables are listed under this category. They may be consumed freely, and as such the portions that you may select are unlimited in quantity.

They are a great source of vitamins, minerals and antioxidants, and a great way to fill you up – so indulge as much as you like. In order to ensure that you obtain your full complement of available nutrients you should eat at least several portions each day. Stir fries, salads, fresh home-pressed juices etc. are a great means of getting a range of these fabulous vegetables each day.

Remember though, that like all foods, if you cook them using any fats or oils, these must be taken from, and limited to, your daily allowance.

They include:

All green leafy vegetables, all green leafy herbs, asparagus, cauliflower, Brussels sprouts, broccoli, courgettes, runner / string beans, mangetout, mushrooms, cucumber, tomato, celery, cress, radishes, peppers, aubergine, artichokes (not Jerusalem!), chicory, bok choy, water chestnuts, bamboo shoots, bean sprouts, onions, garlic, leeks etc.

Starchy Vegetables

The vegetables in this category, as we have already discussed, contain high amounts of starch, and, having higher GI values, are more quickly converted into glucose than non-starchy vegetables. Therefore, these should be limited within your daily food plan.

For the same purposes that refined grains are to be avoided, so are ordinary potatoes – their sugars are released very quickly and can disrupt blood-sugar balance. For this reason, they are not represented within this table.

Starchy Vegetables A typical portion should deliver about 50 calories of energy. All values represent raw weight, unless otherwise specified. If oil or fats are used in cooking, these must be taken as part of the fat allowance for the day.	
Food item	**Amount in a single portion**
Carrots	100 grams
Parsnips	75 grams
Beetroots	100 grams
Pumpkin	200 grams
Squashes (acorn, butternut etc.)	100 grams
Sweet potatoes	50 – 60 grams
Swede	200 grams
Turnips	200 grams
Jerusalem artichokes	75 grams

Fruits

We know that fruits are great sources of nutrients, but their high sugar content means that they should be limited too as part of your food plan. Bananas are excluded from the list, both because they are very high in starches and therefore inappropriate for blood sugar balance, and due to their dampening properties according to traditional Chinese dietetic principles.

Juices are inappropriate, due to the high quantities of sugar-laden fruit required to make a reasonable sized volume of the liquid.

Fruits	
A typical portion should deliver about 80 calories of energy.	
All values represent raw weight, unless otherwise specified.	
If oil or fats are used in cooking, these must be taken as part of the fat allowance for the day.	
Food item	**Amount in a single portion**
Apple	180 grams (about 1 medium sized fruit)
Pear	140 grams (about 1 small sized fruit)
Apricot	165 grams
Peach	200 grams (about 1 large sized fruit)
Nectarine	200 grams (about 2 small sized fruits)
Plum	180 grams (about 3 small-sized or 2 large fruits)
Berries: strawberry, raspberry, blueberry, blackberry, loganberry, black currants, red currants, cranberry etc	100 grams
Melon: cantaloupe, honeydew, galia etc.	200 grams
Water melon	250 grams
Cherry	120 grams
Grape	100 grams
Citrus: orange, grapefruit, tangerine, clementine etc.	150 grams
Pineapple	150 grams
Mango	120 grams
Papaya	150 grams

Pomegranate	100 grams
Passion fruit	80 grams
Guava	100 grams

Nuts and Seeds

Peanuts are omitted from this list as they are considered to be dampening according to traditional Chinese dietetics, so for most people with a weight loss goal are therefore probably inappropriate. Here we are specifically focusing on raw nuts – not the ready roasted and salted varieties, nor those coated in spicy powders or honey etc.

Nuts and Seeds

A typical portion should deliver about 100 calories of energy.

All values represent raw weight, unless otherwise specified.

If oil or fats are used in cooking, these must be taken as part of the fat allowance for the day.

Food item	Amount in a single portion
Almonds	18 grams (approx 15 nuts)
Hazelnuts / Filberts	16 grams (approx 12 nuts)
Cashews	18 grams
Macadamia	13 grams (approx 5 nuts)
Walnut	14 grams (approx 8 nuts)
Pecans	14 grams (approx 10 nuts)
Pistachios	18 grams (approx 25 nuts)
Brazils	14 grams (3-4 nuts)
Sunflower seeds	17 grams
Pumpkin / squash seeds	18 grams
Sesame seeds	18 grams
Flaxseeds / linseeds	18 grams
Nut butters	18 grams (approx 1 tablespoon)
Seed butters	16 grams (approx 1 tablespoon)

Healthy fats

Healthy fats are derived from plant sources, and provide unsaturated fats. I have also included coconut oil, which is a very stable oil for cooking, and, although it is rich in saturated fatty acids, it has been shown to be beneficial to health. Most of these fats are in oil form, BUT where items are especially high in fat content, they may be consumed as the plant-based food from which they are derived.

Healthy fats	
A typical portion should deliver about 40 calories of energy.	
Food item	**Amount in a single portion**
Olive oil	5 grams (about 1 teaspoon)
Nut / seed oils: walnut, sesame etc.	5 grams (about 1 teaspoon)
Flaxseed oil (cold pressed)	5 grams (about 1 teaspoon)
Olives	50 grams (10 small or 5 large / queen olives)
Avocado	25 grams
Mayonnaise (only from a good oil)	5 grams (about 1 teaspoon)
Coconut oil	5 grams (about 1 teaspoon)

A word about drinks

Now we have considered your plan from the food angle, let's look at drinks.

Alcohol, in all its forms - beers, wines and spirits, is a concentrated source of sugars, and rapidly and easily disrupts blood-sugar balance. All types of alcohol should therefore be avoided during your 12 week plan – and minimised thereafter.

Tea and coffee are highly caffeinated. Research has shown that caffeine creates stress in the body, and disturbs the hormonal balances, including insulin and the stress hormones. Caffeine should be definitely avoided during your 12 week plan. Of course, low-caffeine or caffeine-free drinks do not cause the same problems, and therefore may be consumed. If you use decaffeinated products, you should consider the way in which caffeine is removed from such drinks – typically the processes use chemicals that are not optimal in supporting general health and well-being. Think instead about alternatives, such as naturally low or caffeine free varieties, including Rooibosh (Red Bush) tea, green tea, white tea, herbal and fruit teas etc.

Juices may be taken as long as they are made entirely from non-starchy vegetables. Remember that juices made from concentrates are inappropriate, and considered dampening from a traditional Chinese dietetics perspective. Rather they should be fresh-pressed. There is nothing more tasty than a juice made from peppers or tomatoes for example. Experiment to find combinations that you love. Remember that you can add fresh herbs and spices to infuse even more great flavour!

Cordials / squashes / presses etc. should be avoided as they are sweetened. Even low-calorie artificial sweeteners will disrupt your blood sugar. Let's remind ourselves about recent research, which has found that people who regularly drink sugar-free / 'diet' beverages are just as likely to be obese as those who consume the full-sugar alternatives. This is because when the brain registers the sweet flavour of artificial sweeteners it triggers a biochemical response that will disrupt the blood-sugar control mechanisms of our bodies.

Flavoured waters, as long as they are unsweetened may be selected. However, a good quality still or sparkling mineral water is absolutely the ideal choice for your fluid needs. Try a great quality mineral water with a squeeze of natural lemon or lime for a great-tasting and properly hydrating drink! Warm water with a squeeze of lemon or lime is a fabulous way to start your day, and begin your hydration. Remember that water retention is discouraged by drinking water, so for weight and health purposes drinking water makes the perfect choice.

Fine tuning your plan

At this stage, your food plan already incorporates some essential principles for optimum health and weight loss, and you can, of course, use it just as it already is. However, you have the opportunity to fully personalise it, tailoring it precisely to your own health needs.

This can be done in two ways:

First you can assess whether you have any possible commonly-occurring micro-nutrient deficiencies. The questionnaire below will help you to determine any *possible* issues. Remember, only a one to one consultation with a suitably trained professional will give you a totally reliable answer, and I would strongly suggest that you use nutritional supplements only with professional advice and guidance. However, you can at least use this tool to fine tune your food plan – incorporating more of the foods, detailed in the tables provided in Chapter 3, to your best advantage.

To use the questionnaire, simply tick all of the signs and symptoms that apply to you. If you find you have ticked 3 or more in any single category, then pay particular attention to foods containing that specific nutrient. Easy!

Note: Signs and symptoms may fall into more than one category. This highlights the need for a varied balanced diet.

Vitamin A	Night blindness
	Dry rough skin
	Skin disorders
	Frequent colds/respiratory infections
	Slow recovery after illness
	Frequent thrush/cystitis
Vitamin B	Fatigue/sluggishness
	Muscular/general weakness
	Headaches/migraines
	Light-headedness
	Dizziness
	Poor memory/concentration/co-ordination
	Anxiety
	Irritability
	Hair loss/dry hair
	Dry gritty eyes
	Grinding teeth
	Sore/sensitive mouth/lips/tongue
	Geographic tongue
	Dry skin/ skin disorders
	Water retention
Vitamin C	General pain/weakness
	Loss of appetite
	Frequent respiratory infections
	Poor immunity
	Easy bruising
	Raised hair follicles
	Sore bleeding gums

Vitamin D	Hair loss
	Tooth decay
	Limited sun exposure
	Weak/dry/brittle nails
	Bone tenderness/weakness
	Joint pain/inflammation
Vitamin E	Poor circulation in legs
	Hormonal irregularities
	Fertility problems
	Frequent colds
	Poor/slow tissue repair
Vitamin K	Nose bleeds
	Nausea in pregnancy
	Poor bone repair
	Kidney stones
	Poor blood clotting
	Profuse bleeding
Calcium	Muscle cramps
	Weak/dry/brittle nails
	Anxiety
	Depression
	Irritability
	Insomnia
	Sore bleeding gums
	High blood pressure
Chromium	Energy dips
	Anxiety
	Irritability
	Slow tissue repair
	Sweet cravings
	Excessive thirst

Iron	General fatigue
	Heavy periods/blood loss
	Weak/dry/brittle nails
	Dry rough skin
	Sore tongue
	Dry hair
	Apathy/lethargy/listlessness
Magnesium	Apprehension
	Depression
	Apathy/lethargy/listlessness
	Insomnia
	Constipation
	Muscle cramps
	Muscle twitching
	High blood pressure
Manganese	Dizziness
	Memory loss
	Anxiety
	Irritability
	Tooth grinding
	Joint pain
Potassium	Irregular heart beat
	Muscle aches and pains
	Cramps
	Constipation
	Depression
	Headaches
	Confusion
	Extreme thirst
Selenium	Hair loss
	Skin disorders

	Frequent colds
	Frequent respiratory infections
	Muscle weakness
	Muscle spasm/pain
	High blood pressure
Zinc	Poor sense of smell
	Poor sense of taste
	Geographic tongue
	Halitosis
	Stretch marks
	Loss of appetite
Omega-3	Low metabolic rate
	High blood pressure
	Water retention
	Impaired vision
	Impaired learning
	Poor co-ordination
	Poor memory
	Inflammation
	Inflammatory pain

Some of the most important factors pertaining to traditional Chinese dietetics have already been built in to the food tables in this chapter. However, as I have shown you, really fine-tuning your diet according to your own qi profile can be immensely beneficial for your general health and well-being as well as for weight-loss purposes. I cannot encourage you enough to consider this. The second questionnaire, below, should help you to identify some possible issues that you might begin to address by selecting the appropriate foods. Of course, you should ideally consult with a suitably trained, qualified and experienced professional practitioner to help you to determine your own profile. The food tables provided in Chapter 3 will then give you some guidance in what to include or remove from your food plan. The information extracted from them should be used alongside the food categories detailed above.

For example, if you wish to emphasise dampness elimination in your own food plan, you will note that grapes are a good choice, and you may wish to ensure you regularly include grapes as one of your fruit portions. Similarly walnuts would be a great choice as a nut and seed selection, celery fabulous as a regular non-starchy vegetable choice etc.

You still have a hugely varied choice of foods, but with the wisdom borrowed from traditional Chinese dietetics, you can truly fine-tune your own individualised plan.

If you tick 3 or more signs/symptoms in any category, you may benefit from taking the actions shown:	
CATEGORIES	ACTIONS
Dampness Loss of appetite with full feeling Feeling of heaviness, especially in legs and lower body Muzzy headedness Dizzy with muzziness Poor sense of smell/taste Dull grey complexion Puffy/spotty skin Constant or frequent fungal type infection: thrush, cystitis, athletes foot, fungal nail etc. Fatigue with sluggishness Lethargy	Avoid foods listed as damp Incorporate foods listed as damp-resolving
Blood deficiency Dull low-grade headaches Light headedness Trouble getting off to sleep at night Dry hair/eyes Floaters in eyes Sores in corner of mouth/sore lips Pale/sallow complexion Rough dry skin Weak/brittle/dry nails Fatigue	Incorporate blood forming foods

Very light periods	
Blood Stasis Muscle or joint pains that are stabbing in nature Stabbing period pains Clotty menstrual blood Sharp stabbing headaches	Incorporate blood moving foods
Qi deficiency General weakness/fatigue Confusion/poor concentration/indecision Easy bruising Excessive perspiration Low immunity e.g. easily/frequently catching colds and 'bugs' Slow recovery after illness Loss appetite Frequent diarrhoea	Incorporate qi forming foods
Qi Stagnation Poor circulation, especially affecting legs Muscle cramps Muscle spasms/pain Crampy period pains Tightness in shoulders/neck Constipation Nausea/vomiting Belching/hiccups Gastric discomfort Irritability Pre-menstrual Syndrome	Incorporate qi moving foods
Yin deficiency/Excessive heat Feelings of intense heat Heat at night/night sweats Restless tossing and turning at night	Avoid heating foods Incorporate yin forming foods Where high-grade heat exists, incorporate cooling foods

Waking in the night Angry outbursts Redness in eyes Nose bleeds Sore/bleeding gums Sore tongue Halitosis Skin problems characterised by redness Inflammation Hot/inflamed joints	
Yang deficiency/Excessive cold Feelings of extreme cold Cold/chilly sensations Low back pain, not due to injury Weakness in knees Frequent urination Watery stools/diarrhoea Water retention	Avoid cooling foods Incorporate yang-forming foods Where excessive cold exists, incorporate heating foods

Note:

It is vitally important that you do not use these questionnaires as a substitute for consulting a doctor or other suitably qualified healthcare practitioner. Some of the signs/symptoms listed may indicate serious illness, so never rely solely on this information to address health concerns.

Portion selections

Your own energetic needs help you to determine the numbers of portions from each food category. You should always aim to have one portion from each category every day – of course depending upon your qi profile you will need to be careful to avoid those selections that are associated with dampening your qi. By ensuring such a wide cross-section of foods in your daily diet you will optimise the nutrient values of your diet.

In the tables below I have proposed how many portions from each category would be advantageous for you, depending upon the number of calories you need to consume to satisfy your overall metabolic rate. These cover your basic three meals per. day, but on top of those you need to build in 2 snacks – one mid-morning and one mid-afternoon to ensure your blood-sugar balance is optimised, ensuring better body composition, overall health and vitality.

Your snack options may be taken from any of the food categories but are best tailored to meet your daily activities. For example, if you are sitting at your desk on this particular day, choosing high protein, low starch / sugar options, e.g. say oatcakes and a nut butter; or hummus and vegetable crudites made from your non-starchy vegetables such as cauliflower, celery, peppers etc; or a small bean salad; or extra portions of nuts etc. Conversely, if you are enjoying a physically active day, then additional sweet or starchy foods may be appropriate, e.g. additional fruit and nuts, hummus with starchy vegetable crudités such as carrot sticks; an additional grain portion etc.

The amount of calories you should reserve for each snack are also shown in the following table:

Food Categories	Calorific values needed to support overall metabolic rate						
	1100	1200	1300	1400	1500	1600	1700
Complete proteins (150 cals)	1 (or 2 if no dairy selected)	1 (or 2 if no dairy selected)	2	2	2	3	3
Dairy (80 cals)	1 (optional)	1 (optional)	1	1	1	1	1
Wholegrains (100 cals)	1	1	1	1	1	1	1
Pulses (100 cals)	1	1	1	2	2	2	2
Non-starchy vegetables (unlimited)	4 (minimum)	4 (minimum)	4 (minimum)	4 (minimum)	4 (minimum)	4 (minimum)	4 (minimum)
Starchy vegetables (50 cals)	1	1	1	1	1	1	2
Fruit (80 cals)	1	1	1	1	2	2	2
Nuts / seeds (100 cals)	1	1	1	1	1	1	1
Healthy fats (40 cals)	4	4	4	4	4	4	4
Snacks	2 x 160 cals total	2 x 240 cals total	2 x 230 cals total	2 x 230 cals total	2 x 250 cals total	2 x 200 cals total	2 x 250 cals total

Food Categories	Calorific values needed to support overall metabolic rate						
	1800	1900	2000	2100	2200	2300	2400
Complete proteins (150 cals)	3	3	3	3	3	4	4
Dairy (80 cals)	1	1	2	2	2	2	2
Wholegrains (100 cals)	1	1	1	2	2	2	2
Pulses (100 cals)	2	2	2	2	2	2	3
Non-starchy vegetables (unlimited)	5 (minimum)	5 (minimum)	5 (minimum)	5 (minimum)	6 (minimum)	6 (minimum)	6 (minimum)
Starchy vegetables (50 cals)	2	2	2	2	2	2	2
Fruit (80 cals)	2	2	2	2	3	3	3
Nuts / seeds (100 cals)	1	2	2	2	2	2	2
Healthy fats (40 cals)	6	6	6	6	6	6	6
Snacks	2 x 250 cals total	2 x 240 cals total	2 x 260 cals total	2 x 260 cals total	2 x 260 cals total	2 x 200 cals total	2 x 200 cals total

The preceding tables represent highly beneficial combinations of the various food categories, but they can be tweaked if necessary. For example, if on one day you take an extra portion of nut or seeds instead of a portion of legumes it really doesn't matter very much, or if you substitute a fruit portion for a starch vegetable portion it isn't going to do any harm. It is, however, important to avoid substituting categories where they do not represent the same kinds of levels of protein versus carbohydrates. For example, substituting fruit for legumes means you are creating an imbalance between protein-rich and carbohydrate-rich categories. So do take care not to alter the overall proportions of carbohydrates, proteins and fats too much.

Tips for general health

We have already looked at some general guidance in terms of overall health, but let's summarise just a few points here:

- Balance macronutrients in respect of carbohydrates, proteins, fats
- Always eat proteins or fats alongside carbohydrates – never eat carbs without protein or fat to slow down the rate at which the body will convert them to sugar, e.g. have a few nuts or small piece of cheese or natural full-fat yoghurt with fruit, or hummus with an oatcake...
- Consider your daily activities when devising your snacks. i.e.
  - Carbohydrate-based snacks only when undertaking physical activities
  - Protein-based snacks when more sedentary
- Red meat should only be eaten about once each week, as it contains high levels of saturated fats
- The same for most cheeses, though mozzarella, ricotta and feta are less problematic
- Oily fish should be selected about 3 times per. week, or appropriate supplements should be considered for Omega-3 (vegetarians note – this may include an additional portion or two of flax seed oil taken with sea-weed/algae supplements to help the EPA, DHA conversion process)
- Eat 5 times every day – never go for more than 3-4 hours without eating: this will maintain a smoother blood sugar profile
- Stay well-hydrated – water is a vital nutrient too!

When you should eat

So now we have looked in great detail at how much to eat of different types of food, and your plan is looking pretty good!

It's worth thinking a little bit more about the best times of day to eat.

The primary concern here is to promote optimum blood sugar balance, and your plan requires you to eat 5 times each day, at intervals of approximately 3-4 hours. However, within those parameters there is still scope to decide when you should take your larger meals, and when to incorporate smaller snacks. In the main this would depend on when you carry out your main activities of the day.

Let's take a look at Janet's case:

When I met her, Janet had been diagnosed with type 2 diabetes for about 2 years. She is moderately active, and enjoys playing table tennis in the afternoons 3 times each week. Before I saw her she regularly experienced hypoglycaemic episodes after playing. She had developed the habit of taking a snack in readiness for after her game to deal with her hypos, but, nonetheless, as many people experiencing similar episodes will agree, she would still feel slightly unwell even after the immediacy of the low blood sugar had been resolved. My advice to Janet was incredibly simple: why not change her eating patterns on the days she plays table tennis, so that an hour or so before her game she eats some porridge (more specifically the amazing bagsofHEALTH Energy Balance porridge!) to provide her with protein-rich, slow-release carbohydrates to provide her with sufficient energy throughout her afternoon?

Janet then organises her other meals around this activity – ensuring she times her breakfast, and lunch around her porridge 'snack'. This has worked extremely well for her, and Janet hasn't experienced any more hypos following her table tennis sessions.

Hayley's case is also relevant here:

Hayley has type 1 diabetes and, before I met her, was controlling it quite well with insulin. However, Hayley felt she needed to lose weight, was generally fatigued, and a little fearful of her diabetes. As a Phys. Ed. teacher she leads a highly active lifestyle, and did at times experience hypos as a result of her high levels of exercise.

*She embarked on **'the 6 diet'**, and experienced great benefits very quickly: Hayley had significantly reduced her fast-acting insulin from 5 or more shots per. day to just 2 shots within 2 weeks of starting her new eating regime. She was losing weight at exactly the right rate, and she felt more energetic and vital. Her blood sugars were extremely well balanced during the daytime, but she had experienced a couple of hypoglycaemic attacks during the* *night-time.*

This was resolved quickly and easily by adjusting the timing of Hayley's eating plan, and building in a supper – again a small portion of bagsofHEALTH Energy Balance porridge. Hayley has gone on to further reduce her Novorapid to just one shot per. day.

Whilst these cases highlight the need to build individuality into your own plan – tailoring it for your own unique needs and circumstances by tweaking your basic eating schedule – there are still some useful general guidelines that you will find helpful when deciding on meal times. Here we have a wonderful synergy between traditional western and Chinese thinking.

Breakfast like a king

I am sure you are familiar with the old saying:

"Breakfast like a king, lunch like a prince, and dine like a pauper"

In the west, we might simply consider this to be a saying, or even an old wives' tale. However, within traditional Chinese medicine, this saying takes on a whole new relevance. To understand, from a traditional Chinese dietetics perspective, the importance placed upon the timing of meals, we need a brief overview of the meridian system:

There are a total of twelve 'primary' channels, or meridians, within our qi network. Their purpose is to connect up and circulate qi to all parts of the body, to support the various functions of all of the organs, and to provide energy, moisture and nourishment to all the body parts and tissues. Together these twelve primary channels make up one complete circuit, ensuring the flow of qi around all parts of the body. The qi completes one full circuit in each twenty-four hour period, or one day. This means that the qi is at its strongest in each of the channels for a period of two hours, before it leaves to enter the next in the circuit. As we saw in Chapter 3, the main channels involved in digestion are the spleen and stomach channels. So now we can add that for two hours each day, the qi is strongest in the spleen channel, and for the next two hours it is at its strongest in the stomach channel. Twelve hours later, when the flow of qi reaches the opposite side of the circuit, the qi is at its weakest in each of those two channels in turn.

Because the qi flows into and out of each of the channels at the same time in each twenty-four hour period, we can say that there is a 'time' for each channel. The 'time' for each channel indicates when the qi is at its strongest in that channel. There is a 'spleen time', when the qi reaches its peak within the spleen channel; and there is a 'stomach time', when the qi is at its strongest in the stomach channel. When the qi is strong within a channel, the organ related to that channel is most able to fulfil its energetic functions effectively and efficiently. Twelve hours later, when the qi is at its weakest point in that channel, the related organ is least prepared to be able to function well.

This idea of circuitous well-being corresponds very well with our own idea of the 'body clock'. We are quite familiar with the idea that our bodies are programmed to carry out some processes better at certain times of the day – that there is a time to sleep, and a time to wake, a best time for exercise and a best time for work etc. You may be familiar with similar notions of circadian rhythms or bio rhythms? So it is the same with the twenty-four hour flow of qi. It means the body is best able to carry out certain functions at specific times of the day.

Furthermore, we know that if we disturb our body clock, we do not function properly. For example, if we travel across time zones, we often experience jet-lag. Our bodies want to wake at night-time and sleep in the daytime; we may experience disorientation, headaches, and want to eat at strange times. It takes time for our body clocks to adjust to the new time zone, and re-establish a comfortable pattern in which we can function in accordance with the time of day. The twenty-four hour flow of qi explains this phenomenon. When we travel into another time zone we struggle to adapt because our bodies are trying to function when the flow of qi is strongest in the wrong part of the circuit. The flow, just as our body clocks, will adapt, working in harmony with the natural environmental qi – but this adaptation takes time.

Crucially, the 'stomach time' begins at 7:00am each morning when the qi flows most strongly into that channel. It continues until 9:00am, when the flow of qi moves from the stomach channel and into the spleen channel. So begins 'spleen time' at 9:00am each morning. This, of course, means that from 7:00am to 9:00am each morning, the stomach is best able to carry out its functions, and for its part, the spleen functions most effectively between 9:00am and 11:00am each morning.

Thus, our bodies are best able to digest food between 7:00am and 11:00am. Of course, twelve hours later, the qi in the stomach and spleen channels is at its weakest. And so our bodies are least able to digest food between 7:00pm and 11:00pm. And there we have support for our old wives' tale! A basis on which we can agree that breakfast is our most important meal of the day – a time when we can make the best use of our most substantial meal.

By lunchtime, the qi has only just moved on from your spleen channel, and as such the qi available to your stomach and spleen is not too depleted. This means that your body can probably cope with a reasonable lunch. The qi is not as strong as at breakfast time, but it is not yet too weak to cope with the digestive processes. It is such a shame that so many people either skip lunch or have a small and hurried meal to fit in with the daily routine.

By dinner time, or when you take your evening meal – which, for many, is probably also the largest meal of the day – the qi available to your stomach and spleen to aid the digestive processes is at its weakest. Eating a large evening meal overloads the capacity of your stomach and spleen to cope, and impairs their normal functions. No wonder so many people experience indigestion after eating late at night!

As we can see, the usual western pattern of eating is totally inappropriate for getting the best out of your food. What you really need is to make breakfast a main meal time – ensuring the most difficult to digest foods of the day are taken. This meal may include whole grains or protein-based foods, which require the most digestive effort to process. Then you should take a small lunch, ensuring that the foods you choose are a little easier to digest. Small portions of meats, or vegetarian proteins, with lots of vegetables are most suitable. Finally, you should eat only a small amount in the evening. This should ideally be the easiest meal to digest – consisting mainly of vegetables and fruits, with smaller amounts of proteins to ensure you continue to balance your blood sugars. Certainly, the digestive system is not able to cope well with rich meats and heavy proteins during this time.

As much as possible, you should avoid eating after 7:00pm in the evening, when your stomach and spleen are least able to cope with digestion.

As the day progresses, of course to maintain blood sugar balance, it is important to keep our food intake topped up. However, choosing lighter foods later in the day is generally appropriate – unless of course your activity patterns demand more energy at specific times, when it is more appropriate to take measures like those of Janet and Hayley described above.

This practice may require some adaptation, but it will be worth the effort. Your body will have energy at its disposal to get you through the day, and a sense of increased vigour and vitality should quickly become apparent.

If you really are one of the people who simply cannot face food immediately on waking, that is fine – just ensure that you follow the same principles of eating most early in the day, and decreasing the amounts that are consumed as the day progresses.

Onwards and upwards

You now have everything you need to make a great start. You have all the knowledge to support your journey, and hopefully to provide you with the motivation to get going and keep going. Your journey on **'the 6 diet'** can only be really beneficial!

You have a well thought out plan, tailored specifically to your own needs and to meet all your own health and well-being goals. There really is no stopping you now! Or is there?

If only life was always as simple, straight forward and supportive as **'the 6 diet'**. But, there's always a but! Life throws us some interesting curve balls now and again!

The chapters from this point forward are designed to help you understand and cope with all the issues that might impact on your journey. Change is thrilling and exciting and challenging. There are certainly challenges involved in any lifestyle change. What we will learn next is that food isn't the only thing that has a great impact on blood sugar control. Other lifestyle factors, notably stress and exercise, exert huge effects on our blood sugars, so now you know what to do to get started, let's take a look at what to do next!

Chapter 5:

Other lifestyle factors

The role of stress

Optimum digestion and weight management, maybe surprisingly, are not just matters of eating the right foods or the right quantities of foods. Stress can significantly disrupt the way in which our bodies process foods. That said, it's worth understanding exactly what is stress. Well, according to the International Stress Management Association (ISMA) UK, it can be defined as follows:

"The adverse reaction people have to excessive pressures or
Other types of demand placed on them"

What this means is that stress is a bodily reaction – it comes from within us rather than being something imposed upon us.

We all need a stress response

We hear many negative messages about stress and the way it impacts on our health that it's easy to overlook the fact that we absolutely need a biochemical response to stress. In fact, our very lives could depend on it!

On a daily basis we are protected from potential disaster by a number of hormones, which are very quickly released in times of danger. Adrenaline is one of these hormones, and serves to give us almost superhuman, though very temporary, capacities to get out of danger. This response is commonly known as the 'fight or flight' response. It is rooted in our evolutionary past, and is designed to protect us from the proverbial sabre-toothed tigers that once threatened our survival. At times when our actual physical survival is threatened, there is no better response to have on our side. This surge of vital hormones is the force responsible for amazing feats such as mothers lifting cars off their trapped children and for firemen heroically running into blazing houses to save endangered victims. It imbues us with heroism and courage at times when we are called upon to protect and defend the lives and values we cherish. Crucially, when the danger has passed, the hormones subside and our bodies return to a more normally balanced biochemistry.

When stress becomes toxic

The problem we face today is that although life has dramatically changed, our bodies have not evolved at the same rate. Today's equivalents of the sabre-toothed tigers are more likely to be things like the rush hour traffic, the threat of missing a deadline, having an argument with a friend, family member or colleague. Nonetheless, these stresses trigger the same ancient activation of our fight or flight system as if our physical survival was threatened.

On a daily basis, toxic stress hormones flow into our bodies for reasons that pose no real threat to our physical survival. In other words, the effects of emotional stress are exactly the same, in biochemical terms, as those of physical threat, even though they are not entirely appropriate. Our bodies don't recognise the difference between physical danger and emotional stress – they behave in exactly the same way. The problem is that the emotional stresses that we typically encounter are not over as quickly as they begin. Difficult life circumstances tend to last longer than the danger of a prowling wild beast.

Our bodies are well geared up to cope with these powerful stress hormones on a short-term basis, but we cope far less well when our bodies are flooded with them for long periods of time. Retaining these chemicals can establish a situation with some damaging consequences! When the fight or flight response continues in the long term, our bodies enter the 'adaptive phase', with physical manifestations as follows:

- Adrenal glands release other stress hormones, one of which is Cortisol
- Chronically high levels of these hormones give rise to high blood pressure & high cholesterol
- Stomach secretes too much acid
- Sex hormones diminish
- Brain becomes starved of glucose impairing mental ability
- Immune system is under pressure and therefore prone to infections & illness

Long term stress is associated with a whole range of symptoms, including:

- Digestive problems
- High blood pressure
- Increased heart rate and cholesterol
- Increased blood sugar levels – crucial when considering the effect of stress on diabetes!
- Insomnia
- Irritability
- Depression

- Headaches
- Overeating
- Fatigue

For **'the 6 diet'** purposes, we need to concentrate on cortisol. In the adaptive phase cortisol becomes powerfully involved.

It isn't just stress that causes us to produce cortisol - fasting, eating and exercising also flood our bodies with this hormone. Typically, we have a peak of cortisol each morning, which declines as the day progresses. It plays a vital part in regulating our energy, and is responsible for tapping into our bodies' own reserves. For example, it determines whether we can best meet our energy demands by selecting to convert carbohydrates, proteins or fats: it can tap into our own fat stores or it may use our own lean tissues as a source of nutrients depending upon the circumstances.

What this means in **'the 6 diet'** terms is that cortisol can affect and even alter our body composition.

***Yes, that's right – stress hormones can alter body composition**!*

Sometimes that may be a beneficial change, but conversely it can be an adverse change.

In periods of long-term stress, when body tissues are exposed to high levels of cortisol for extended amounts of time, adverse cellular and tissue alterations may occur. These high levels of cortisol cause changes in the way that fat is stored and deposited around the body. Essentially, cortisol becomes the decision maker – charged with determining how to meet the body's energy demands: should it take energy from our fat stores, or by breaking down and converting our own healthy lean tissues? Typically it decides on the latter – it generates glucose from the lean tissues within our body. Any excess glucose is removed from the blood, processed as usual by the liver, and so often is stored as abdominal fat. In this way, the body begins to swap its lean tissues for abdominal fat: fat that becomes concentrated in the abdomen creating the so-called apple shape. As we have covered in earlier chapters of this book, this is the pattern of body fat that is linked with diabetes, heart disease and other serious illnesses. So, if left unchecked stress can either lead to or increase abdominal obesity and encourage the development of type 2 diabetes and all the other associated health risks that we have previously discussed.

As shown in the list above, cortisol has a direct impact on blood sugar levels. Under the influence of cortisol, blood sugar levels can rise significantly, regardless of your eating plan.

Let's revisit Hayley (the same lady whose case we briefly looked at previously):

During her 12 week plan, Hayley experienced one highly stressful week. She reported that, although she continued to stick closely to her eating plan, her blood sugar levels were temporarily elevated. Having enjoyed blood glucose levels of 6 – 7 for a few weeks Hayley suddenly found her levels rose sharply into double figures again. As soon as her stress was resolved her blood glucose levels fell again to their previous single figures. Hayley no longer takes her body for granted during stressful times, and has learned to build in proper relaxation techniques to her daily routine.

As well as causing havoc with blood sugar levels, high levels of cortisol are connected with appetite disturbances: simply put, it makes us crave sweet and fatty foods and increases our appetite by interacting with the hormones that regulate hunger and satiety: leptin!

So there we have it – stress hormones can disturb our appetites, mess with our metabolism, and cause us to store body fat in the most unhealthy manner. There is a direct causal link between stress, weight gain, poor blood sugar control and an unhealthy body composition!

Coping strategies

Of course, what this all means is that we need to develop strategies for dealing with stress. This is not only vitally important for our general health, but even more so when we are trying to manage blood sugars and weight. Stress is perfectly capable of interfering with our agendas for health, appearance and well-being through the interaction of cortisol with our dietary intake, and internal nutrient stores.

Achieving your ideal body, therefore, involves more than simply ensuring you make appropriate and beneficial food choices. It means taking care of yourself in a much wider sense – emotionally and spiritually as well as physically!

Managing emotional stress is a whole other topic, and much more than we can deal with properly in this book. Nonetheless, I have included some aspects in Section 6, which I hope you may find helpful and uplifting!

What we can usefully discuss here, however, is the impact that exercise can have on moderating the effects of cortisol. The right exercise has been shown to have a beneficial effect on reducing cortisol levels and therefore cortisol effects.

But, first we need to dispel some myths about exercise as well as nutrition. So here goes!

Not all exercise is beneficial!

Indeed, the wrong types of exercise can actually create more stress in the body and therefore elevate cortisol and its harmful effects.

So, let's take a brief look at **'the 6 diet'** approach to exercise!

'the 6 diet' approach to exercise

As you may have guessed by now, **'the 6 diet'** dictates that there is no one-size-fits-all to any aspect of health or well-being. Indeed, the same is true of exercise!

Just as some of our inherited 'wisdoms' about food turn out to be no more than myths, so the idea that any exercise has to be good for us is another myth that **'the 6 diet'** aims to dispel!

Some exercise can be extremely damaging to your health. Because the words 'health' and 'fitness' so often live side-by-side in the same phrase we may be fooled into thinking that they amount to one and the same thing. Nothing could be further from the truth. Physical fitness is so often achieved at the expense of health, and it takes real expertise to achieve both together.

When exercise causes physical stress!

Pushing our bodies to their limits causes physical stress. An article in Time magazine summarises this problem:

> "For most people, regular exercise is associated with cardiovascular health. But doctors have long noted a troubling tendency among the ultra-fit: an athlete has a greater chance than the average person of suddenly dropping dead...
>
> According to the International Olympic Committee, that rate is about three times higher than in the normal population."

Of course, when our bodies perceive that physical stress, it responds in the usual manner – it sets up the fight or flight response. The links between exercise and stress are so well known we even adopt the term 'adrenaline junkies' for those who are addicted to stretching their bodies to levels of achievement beyond their normal capacities. Now, remembering that stress hormones cause us to achieve short-term superhuman powers, it's easy to see why it can feel good to have them surging through our bodies –

hence dedicated athletes can feel really grim without their daily 'fix' of adrenaline.

It's hard to believe that exercise can cause stress – and the physical chaos that comes with it – after all it's something that we are supposed to find beneficial and even enjoyable!

When exercise causes you to be fat!

If it's hard to believe that exercise can cause stress, it's probably even harder to believe that inappropriate exercise can actually make you fat?

But **'the 6 diet'** tells us that too is true!

During acute exercise bouts - that is fast and furious and infrequent sessions - cortisol levels become elevated because your body perceives stress.

If you mix a lot of strenuous exercise with an already stressed mental or emotional life, the result is even more cortisol production.

As the cortisol levels increase, there is a greater tendency for you to store fat specifically in your abdomen. People with excessive abdominal fat may believe they need to work out harder and more often. However, although they may lose some weight, they will disappointingly not necessarily lose abdominal fat. In fact, they may even accumulate more!

As crazy as it seems, if you have been working out and feel like you are doing everything right and yet still cannot shift your abdominal fat, you may be overdoing it. Although exercise is an important factor in healthy weight loss, the wrong kind of exercise for certain people may actually be preventing them from losing fat! In fact inappropriate exercise may be the cause of the fat!

When exercise depletes strength

It may not intuitively make sense to think that you can lose physical strength as a result of exercise but cortisol can actually stimulate the breakdown of muscle and other tissue to satisfy your immediate energy needs. As you struggle to work out harder and harder, more and more cortisol is released, and your body responds by breaking down its own muscle and lean tissues for fuel - meaning you lose weight and strength but not fat!

Quite simply – too much or over-taxing exercise makes no sense at all from a health perspective and can be counterproductive in assisting weight loss or for improving body composition!

Effects of exercise on blood sugar control

Exercise has a direct impact on blood sugar balance. Most of the time, as long as the exercise is appropriate, moderate, and not creating a stress response, this is a beneficial effect. As such, exercise is being increasingly promoted for type 2 diabetes. It is now thought that in addition to its cardiovascular benefits, exercise can improve glycaemic control by increasing tissue sensitivity to insulin. In addition to this highly beneficial effect, the muscles initially use glucose in the muscle and later convert muscle glycogen to glucose to provide energy. These two factors, i.e. increased insulin sensitivity and take-up of glucose by the muscles, work together to lower blood sugar levels.

For short bursts of exercise, such as a quick sprint to catch the bus, the muscles and the liver can release stores of glucose for fuel. With continued moderate exercising, the muscles take up glucose at up to 20 times the normal rate. This helps lowers blood sugar levels significantly, so care has to be taken to prevent hypoglycaemic episodes. Even light activities — such as housework, gardening or being on your feet for extended periods — can lower your blood sugar level. The body mechanisms do help to prevent hypos: because the glucose levels fall, at the same time insulin levels may drop in anyone not taking insulin so the risks of too low blood sugar is moderated at least.

Problems, however, can occur with strenuous exercise – the kind that causes a stress response. Because the body recognises intense exercise as a stress and releases stress hormones that tell your body to increase available blood sugar to fuel your muscles, intense exercise can have the opposite effect and actually temporarily increase your blood glucose levels. This is especially true for many people with diabetes, and especially true if intense exercise is combined with emotional stress, which together create the causes for raising blood sugar instead of lowering it!

In terms of blood sugar control, and in the treatment of diabetes, to get the best from your exercise regime, here are some sensible considerations:

- Check your blood sugar level
  - before, during and after exercise, especially if you take insulin or medications. This will help you to monitor the effects of your exercise on your blood sugar levels, to prevent, or detect possible hypoglycaemic episodes, or indeed to identify where blood sugar levels rise!
- Stay hydrated
  - it is crucial to drink plenty of water while exercising because dehydration can adversely affect blood sugar levels.
- Be prepared

o   always have a small snack with you during exercise in case your blood sugar drops too low.

🎗 Adjust your diabetes treatment plan as needed

o   adjust your food intake before exercise to make sure you have slow release nutrients to last through your work out.

o   if you take insulin, you may need to adjust your insulin dose before exercising or wait a few hours to exercise after injecting insulin.

Using exercise with 'the 6 diet'

For those with particular sporting goals, stress – both physical and emotional – is an occupational hazard to be dealt with. However this is a specialist area outside of our focus – so let's leave the problems of athletic burn-out to the experts!

For those of us who wish to use exercise to our greatest benefit – that is to improve our appearance, health and vitality in the most sensible way – here are some things to bear in mind:

🎗 Where strenuous or arduous exercise can cause stress, progressive exercise gives your body the ability to adapt so that the related stress hormones are moderated rather than becoming unduly elevated. This means that regular, low impact, steady and gentle exercise is much more likely to help you to achieve your goals. Key considerations are:

o   Low impact workouts involving walking, cycling, swimming

o   Regularity – say 3 – 5 times per. week

o   Manageable lengths – say 20 -60 minutes per. session

🎗 On an emotional level exercise has to be fun. When it becomes a chore, causes pain or discomfort, or is otherwise not enjoyable it becomes a source of emotional stress – and we now know what that means! So choosing a form of exercise that gives you a sense of enjoyment is absolutely the most beneficial FOR YOU. Whatever appeals to you, within some sensible parameters, is best for you - because it will not only provide physical benefits but will be a way for you to combat other stressors in your life.

o   If you prefer company then choose an activity with a social aspect – maybe dancing or a team activity.

o   If you have a competitive streak, then choose a sport that allows you to indulge it – but keep it within sensible limits!

o   If you like solitude then there is plenty of scope for you to take off alone and immerse yourself into the moment.

- Exercising outdoors can be an excellent stress reducer and as such it is a great way to reduce cortisol production.
- Relaxation exercises can be really valuable. Given that stress is a major factor of cortisol, stress reducing exercises will help lower it. Yoga, Pilates, Tai Chi, Qi Gung etc. all involve meditative breathing work, and as such are all great examples of relaxing types of exercise, whilst still providing really useful physical exertion.

Rather than increasing the intensity of your exercise in a futile battle to get rid of abdominal fat, try to reduce the intensity of the exercise, and look to find a solution to controlling your stress. Amazingly your fatigue, weakness, and soreness should begin to shrink away, and you'll be more likely to achieve the great look and feel that you desire.

The right exercise will really help you to optimise your body composition, bodily appearance, performance and vitality to get the very best out of your life. Of course, by improving your body composition, you also increase your BMR, so that eventually you can get away with the occasional carbohydrate indulgence!

Chapter 6:

Living in the real world

Social eating

Any specific food regime is perfectly controllable in your home environment. You plan your meals, you shop, you cook, you eat. Simple! You are in control.

Of course, it isn't always quite so straightforward when someone else has the responsibility for feeding you. Whether it's dining with friends or eating out, you'll find that it isn't always possible to stick 100% to your plan, despite your best intentions and efforts.

Let's take a look at some of the challenges and, more importantly, solutions to social eating.

Eating out

In our modern world, we are blessed with the opportunity to choose from a wide selection of foods and cuisines when eating out. Some are healthy, and some aren't. Some will support **'the 6 diet'** principles, some won't.

The crux of both the problem and solution is choice! Your food plan gives you plenty of scope to eat out – it incorporates every food group, and in essence is adaptable to any type of cuisine. It is the quantities of each food category that may restrict your choices, as not all restaurant food items are based on the sound thinking underpinning **'the 6 diet'**.

Let's look together at a few examples:

Pizza /pasta

These food items typically consist of a highly refined carbohydrate base, and a selection of toppings. It is rare to find a good quality wholegrain pasta or pizza-base, and even if you do it will be made using wheat grain. If you are able to find a restaurant serving an appropriate type of grain you'll need to be very careful about your portion control. Typical serving sizes will exceed a single portion size as defined within **'the 6 diet'** plan, so do ensure that you take proper account of quantities. For those looking to avoid wheat-based products, clearly this is an inappropriate selection.

Toppings should be carefully selected according to how they contribute to **'the 6 diet'** plan. Vegetables are ideal, and you can freely enjoy tomatoes, peppers, aubergine, courgettes, mushrooms etc. Simply take care with the highly processed ingredients and high levels of saturated fats delivered by other choices: cheese, ham, pepperami / pepperoni, salami, creamy sauces etc.

- **Sandwiches, panini, baguettes, wraps etc.**

    The same considerations apply as for pizza and pasta dishes. You may find a great wholegrain, even wheat-free bread, but take care with your portion control. Also watch out for appropriate fillings. Salad vegetables, roasted vegetables, hummus, egg, chicken, fish etc. can all be enjoyed as part of **'the 6 diet'** plan. Take care with fillings that are highly processed or contain high levels of saturated fats: cheese, bacon, ham, roast pork etc.

- **Tortillas, tacos, pancakes, crepes etc.**

    Again – the same considerations apply! Though fajitas can be a good choice – the fillings are typically ideal, consisting of stir-fried vegetables, chicken or beef – offering you the opportunity to apply your own limitations on the amount or tortilla, soured cream etc. that you add to them.

- **Indian / Pakistani / Bangladeshi / Sri Lankan Cuisines**

    You should typically find a reasonable selection of foods that fit in well with **'the 6 diet'** plan. Tomato-based sauces as opposed to creamy sauces work quite well. If traditional ghee is used in cooking you probably don't have to worry about the kind of fats used in cooking – though the quantities may be beyond your daily allowance. A good dry curry – typified by tandoori baked dishes – is great. Just don't be tempted to overindulge in the accompanying carbohydrate dishes. Rice, chapattis, rotis, naan breads etc. should be kept within your portion limits.

- **Thai / Chinese / Malaysian Cuisines**

    These also can offer appropriate food selections that meet **'the 6 diet'** principles. Eastern cuisines often include healthy stir-fried dishes, though care needs to be applied in the selection of sauces and accompanying carbohydrates in the same way as applies with Indian meals.

- **Mediterranean (Italian, Greek, Spanish etc.) Cuisines**

    Pizzas and pastas aside, there are some fabulous selections available which generally meet **'the 6 diet'** principles. Fish, vegetables and salads, olives, healthy olive oils, feta cheeses, abound in Mediterranean dishes and can easily be built into your daily plan. Paellas, risottos and other high-carbohydrate dishes, however, should be approached with caution – small portions pose few problems, but it can be easy to exceed your portion sizes with these dishes.

- **Middle Eastern and North African (Turkish, Lebanese, Moroccan, Israeli, Arabic etc.) Cuisines**

    Again, these cuisines offer a plethora of fabulous foods: hummus, aubergine-based dips, pulses, vegetables, salads, fish, meats etc. all easily fit into **'the 6 diet'** plan. Take care with the pitta bread portion sizes, and away you go!

🍲 French Cuisine

Generally based on simple and rustic ingredients, such as great quality meats, fish and vegetables, many French dishes pose few problems. An alpine cheese fondue with bread to dip clearly stretches the point but think more in terms of a cassoulet, or a simple steak with haricot vert, mussels cooked in a Provencal style sauce etc. to see how this cuisine can fit **'the 6 diet'** framework. Avoid the potatoes and limit the French breads and you'll be able to stay 'on-plan'.

Dining with friends and acquaintances

Close friends will of course be supportive of your diet plan, and hopefully it is easy to discuss your dietary needs with them.

Accepting an invitation to dine with someone that you don't know very well might limit your ability to control your food choices. If that's the case, you can only do your best to dine within your plan. Think food categories, portion sizes etc. and then settle back and enjoy your evening!

And to follow?

Of course, you will have spotted that I haven't yet addressed the issues of dessert or alcohol or coffee! These are often the things that we struggle with when dining out. Avoiding them at home is easy, but all restaurants, and even our friends, will offer an appetising selection to tempt your palette. This is where our relationships with food come to the fore. Of course some of us have no difficulty in controlling our urges, maybe these things simply don't tempt us anyway. But if you are one of the people who will struggle to resist then you'll need to adopt a strategy to help you avoid or limit inappropriate food choices. And remember, it is a choice – it's your choice!

For example - if you really cannot find satisfaction in a cup of green tea instead of a creamy cappuccino in your favourite coffee bar then why torture yourself? Make a case to find a new favourite juice bar and discover the delights of a fabulous and tasty vegetable juice! Redefining your sense of a 'treat' can be an exciting exploration. Think about this logically – how can a treat be something that has a detrimental effect? Why not consider a treat as something that benefits your body?

Essentially it all boils down to your relationships with food.

The next section is especially for you!

Our relationships with food

Change is difficult

OK then. You have a much better understanding of how your own body works; you have masses more knowledge about nutrition; you have a plan; you have a lifestyle strategy; you know how to cope when you don't have full control in the real world. What can prevent you from succeeding to achieve your ideal body, fabulous appearance, great bodily health and performance?

Well, if you can generally see food as fuel: purely and simply as a physical solution to meet your body's needs – then nothing. If indeed this is the case for you, there is nothing now preventing your success.

It's likely however, that this is not the case. Compliance with dietary change is recognised in the medical world as a huge problem. Many clinical trials have been undertaken to try to establish the best ways to persuade people, even those with serious medical needs, to incorporate and adhere to dietary change.

It all boils down to our relationships with food. Very few of us do truly see food simply as a form of fuel. Instead we have particular associations and attachments to different foods that resonate so strongly with us emotionally and spiritually that the mere physical benefits we get from food pale into a much lesser significance.

Establishing long term, lasting changes can be a real challenge. I know this too, and there is no intention of pretending otherwise. Pretending there is no issue is no way to find the solution!

I really want you to be the very best version of you – and if that's what you want for yourself too, then I am here to support you. So let's take a closer look at some of the issues.

Not all nourishment comes from food

As touched upon earlier, traditional Chinese wisdom, according to some writers, says *we only obtain about 25% of our nourishment from food*. This possibly comes as a big surprise. After all, our western scientific understanding of nutrition boils everything down to a simple equation of nutrients in = results out! If this were truly the case our medical establishments would not be undertaking so much research in order to fulfil the need to find resolutions to the problems of compliance with dietary advice and change! Of course eating has an emotional aspect!

We cannot survive simply by meeting the basic physical need for food and drink. That's because we are not merely physical beings. We are much, much more than that. We are hugely complex beings, combining the physical, the emotional and the spiritual. To ensure our holistic well-being, we also need to nourish the emotional and spiritual aspects of ourselves. It is acknowledged in traditional Chinese philosophies, as well as other Eastern traditions, that about 75% of our nourishment has to be obtained from emotional and spiritual sources. We have an absolute need to satisfy the emotional and spiritual aspects of our being. By the way – in our context the words 'emotional' and 'spiritual' do not mean 'religious'!

In its entirety, this is a huge subject, and I could not possibly hope to do it justice within a single chapter of a book. However, we do need to spend some time on this because it relates very closely with our emotional attitudes regarding food. So often we confuse our needs for emotional and spiritual nourishment with our bodies' needs for physical nutrition, with the result that we seek them both from the same source – food! We develop such strong emotional attachments to particular foods that we experience mental pain if they are removed from us.

Test yourself! To what do you turn when you feel the need for comfort? Celebration? A 'pick-me-up'? The language that we use around food betrays the fact that so often the answer is food or drink. We actually talk about 'comfort food'; we consider some foods to be a 'treat' or 'party food' etc. Of course, we all have different ideas of what constitutes 'comfort food' or a 'treat' – but most of us will indeed identify with the concept! Our problems generally begin when we confuse food with more appropriate sources of emotional and spiritual nourishment.

Essentially, we all need love, respect, friendship, physical touch from other human beings, job satisfaction, emotional security – the list is potentially endless – in order to live well. Some of these things are needed quite simply to enable us to survive. Without emotional and spiritual nourishment we are as empty shells, and cannot hope to achieve lasting health or well-being. Therefore, we all need to find deep pleasure from sources other than food. As we are all unique individuals, we will all find our pleasure in different ways and from different things. It may be from the relationships we share with others: with our family and loved ones; from the bonds we make with friends; parenthood; or through religious practices, and our relationships with our various gods – though do not think this is all I am meaning when I talk about spiritual nourishment! We may experience deep pleasures from our pastimes: a good book; listening to music; walking in the countryside; fishing; tending the garden, etc. Most of us can identify something in our lives from which we can derive great pleasure. Alternatively, we can obtain nourishment from simple activities such as receiving a massage, meditation, relaxation, watching the sunrise or sunset, counting the stars in the clear night sky, sitting in a beautiful garden, listening to flowing water. Again the possibilities are boundless, and limited only by our time and imagination. But, in short, this nourishment is obtained from the relationships we make within our world – with other people, our environment, our spiritual experiences etc.

Food is *not* love

We are often led to believe that fat people are jolly. How rarely this is true! Almost on a daily basis the celebrity who once insisted that she or he was happy to be fat reveals the new, slimmer results of their latest 'miracle diet'. We watch the repeated yo-yo attempts of those in the lime-light as they struggle between overweight and svelte in a now familiar cycle.

How often deeply painful emotional issues lie buried in folds of body fat – evidence that the emotional and spiritual nourishment for an overweight or obese individual is lacking. People deprived of love, contentment, satisfaction and happiness commonly find consolation in food, in an attempt to nourish their emotional and spiritual selves using physical food.

Sadly, for some people, even though they may have a strong desire to lose weight, their relationship with certain foods is so vital to them, that to remove a favourite food may create a deep sense of deprivation. And so we come to the crux of the matter that I want to cover in this chapter. Our emotional relationships with food.

Guilt

We too often tend to think about food in terms of good and bad. Some foods are good for us, and we are virtuous if we eat them. Some foods are bad for us, and we are virtuous if we refuse them. Please let me reiterate: generally speaking, inflammatory foods aside, there are no good foods, and there are no bad foods. Essentially, there are just foods! They may or may not be appropriate for us at that time depending upon our health and lifestyle factors. Certainly, whether we need to lose weight or not, it is likely we need to change our relationships with food. Instead of considering intrinsic moral goodness, or otherwise, of food, we need to recognise it as a means to satisfy *our energetic needs*. If the energetic property of a particular food will benefit us it is appropriate. If not, then we may think that the food, at least at that time, is inappropriate. Food is a fuel, and it should be used to meet our physical needs rather than our emotional and spiritual needs. If only it were that simple!

The fact remains that as individuals we all have an emotional and spiritual history, and our relationships with foods are often a matter of that history. As adults, we possibly have already formed some emotional attachment to a particular food, and would be quite loath to give it up entirely. Maybe there is a food that helps us to get through this life. It may be any food or drink that has some happy connotation. And who is to judge us for it? Rather we have to find our own ways to manage our emotional associations with food. Often we can change our perspectives by understanding their roots. If we are honest about what is lacking in our emotional and spiritual lives we can possibly meet the need in some other way and, though we may occasionally slip, reduce our reliance on our favourite food. If you are absolutely not ready to give up a favourite food, then do yourself one big favour. Stop feeling guilty about it!

If, as we eat, we experience guilt, it cannot be said that we are eating in a relaxed frame of mind. Remember, from the traditional Chinese dietetics perspective, the energetic spleen and stomach are both injured by mental exertion when eating. Therefore, if you decide to eat, then do so with pleasure. Your spleen and stomach will process the food much better if you enjoy your food, and are relaxed about doing so.

In much the same way, take away the same message if you do indeed embark on adopting the weight loss aspects of **'the 6 diet'** approach. And I use the word 'if'. We live in a media-led culture. We are constantly bombarded with images of near-anorexic bodies. This is not ideal! Nor would I encourage anyone to embark upon a weight-loss diet unless their aim is to achieve safe, effective, and healthy weight-loss, within a framework of seeking overall health and well-being. This applies equally to both men and women.

Be honest with yourself about your motivation to change. If your motivation is sincere, you will be successful. Accept yourself entirely, and be motivated by your own needs and wants. It's OK if you do not want the same as others.

You are a unique individual, and your wants and needs are uniquely valid and valuable.

Now, all that said, if you have already developed type 2 diabetes, or have been diagnosed as being insulin resistant and on your way to developing type 2 diabetes, I really hope your motivation to change is heightened; for your own sake. You have now been brought face-to-face with the consequences of you previous dietary and lifestyle habits. The results are not good are they? You, as much as anyone, can see the need to make real changes.

In my clinical experience I see so many people fearful of their diagnosis and ready to make that change. That's great! However, I also see some people who despite all that are still not ready to make changes – I am thinking about the man who insisted he could not give up bacon sandwiches every day for breakfast, nor his three pints of beer three times each week; or the lady who insisted she could never get through her day without several cups of tea with milk and sugar. I choose, and wisely so I think, not to work with people who haven't yet made a strong commitment to change for their own sake. Why? It's simple. If people cannot commit to change for their own sakes, even in the face of a fearsome diagnosis, they certainly won't make changes for the sake of anyone or anything else, and they will be doomed to failure. A failure reinforces negativity for healthy eating and lifestyle, which will potentially put them off committing to change again in the future. It's so much better to encourage them to work to find a motivation to change, and only to embark on a life-long new approach when they have put everything in place to help them succeed!

Blame and responsibility

When first discussing diet with my clinic patients, I am often faced with some who, recognising that their idea of a 'healthy balanced diet' has contributed to a state of ill-health, blame themselves. Similarly, if having read this book you have any sense of blame for your diet thus far – stop. You are not to blame. You have simply done what you thought correct in the light of previous dietary education and your life experiences.

You can, however, take responsibility for your nourishment from now on. Blame and responsibility are entirely different beasts. **'the 6 diet'** empowers you, through the education that it provides, to take responsibility for your food choices, now and for life.

There will be times when you are unable to avoid inappropriate foods, and have limited access to beneficial foods. You may be invited to dine out or with friends. You may be on holiday. Whatever the circumstance, it is unlikely that you will never be faced with less-than-optimal foods again. Also, as we have already discussed, overweight and obesity often hide emotional needs. These will not be magically released or cease to be. Overweight people need nourishment, not starvation and punishment. Even when genuinely trying to lose weight, we may experience a real emotional need for our favourite food. Real deprivation is as harmful to the process of digestion as eating the forbidden fruit. If you experience a real need, then satisfy it. If you occasionally eat inappropriate foods, then do so with pleasure.

All the way through this book you have read the term 'avoid' not 'eliminate'. However, if you are serious about your intentions to lose weight, or otherwise to benefit your health, beware that you do not use this as an excuse to continue to regularly enjoy inappropriate foods, and continue in an unhealthy attitude towards some foods.

Remember, you now have the education, knowledge and understanding to manage your food choices every day for life!

Because you're worth it!

Imagine a kitchen (a). In the kitchen is a cook. The cook is surrounded by fresh, organic foods – the best. The cook carefully and lovingly takes time to prepare and cook a meal. It is carefully presented, on a lovely china plate, which has been pre-warmed. The meal is eaten quietly and peacefully and the food is savoured and appreciated. All this is done with due regard to the alchemical ritual that is dining (we'll come on to that shortly!).

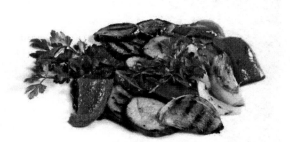

Imagine another kitchen (b). In it is a cupboard. The cupboard is full of ready meals, processed foods, tinned foods. These have all been prepared in a factory quickly and cheaply for – let's admit it – profit. A tin is opened, the contents are heated without much care or attention, probably in a microwave oven, and eaten quickly straight from the dish they were cooked in. The TV is on, and there is a loud argument taking place in the soap opera that is showing.

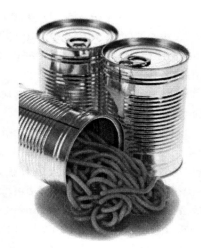

If you were to receive one of the meals, which would you prefer? The one from kitchen (a), or the one from kitchen (b).

It's amazing isn't it, how simply imagining these two scenarios elicits very different responses? Your mind really embraces the first scene, and probably firmly rejects the second?

Hopefully you would choose the meal prepared in kitchen (a) – just the thought of it naturally lifts the spirits and you can already feel that meal doing good things for your body and mind. Our bodies are amazing – they will respond in the same way to something imagined as they will to something real – but that's another book too! Suffice to say then, that the affects you are now imagining are exactly the same as though you were placed in those situations in real life.

Already the alchemy is beginning to work!

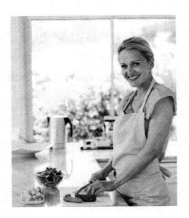 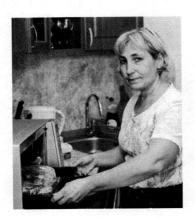

So, which more closely resembles your own kitchen, and your own cooking habits? Are you an enthusiastic cook with a healthy glowing appearance, or are your fast and furious microwave meals giving you that typical grey puffy damp appearance? If it's the latter, well bravo for your honesty: but now it's time to make some changes!

Food represents the ultimate relationship between our environment and ourselves. What do I mean by that?

Let's use our imagination again to place ourselves in two environments. In the first we are sitting on a beach: the sky is blue; the sea is calm and the waves are gently lapping onto clean, warm, golden sands; the air is clean and fresh. In the second we are sitting in a lay-by next to a motorway: the air is full of petrol and diesel fumes; the traffic noise is deafeningly loud; the ground is covered in discarded cigarette waste. OK, so which environment do you wish to be in?

So here's what I mean when I say that food is the ultimate in our relationship with our environment. Usually we find ourselves in our environment. But with food, we take a part of our environment, and actually put it inside our bodies. Its energy interacts with our own, and there is a result. Think about it for a moment: from babyhood to adulthood and beyond, the only resources that your body has to draw upon to physically grow, develop and mature, is the food you eat, the fluids you drink, the air you breathe, and the mental attitudes towards yourself that you decide to adopt. So, just as you wouldn't really want to sit in a dirty, neglected, unhealthy environment for too long, why would you want to put a product from an unhealthy environment inside your body? Yet that is exactly what so many people do the majority of the time!

In taking the responsibility for your choices, **'the 6 diet'** urges you to seek to ensure the result is the best possible. You are indeed worth the best.

We are all indeed worthy of the food from kitchen (a), so why do we tend more towards creating kitchen (b) in our own homes? Time? Pressure? Lifestyle?

Digestion is a magical, alchemical process. Eating is essentially a ritual, and should be honoured as such.

If you eat truly good quality food, prepared and cooked with loving care; if you honour the ritual, dine in the quiet contemplative manner preferred by the energetic stomach and spleen; and if you recognise that you deserve the best – then already you are doing so much for your emotional and spiritual nourishment. You have already promoted the alchemical ritual of dining beyond a mere 25% contribution to your physical, emotional and spiritual well-being.

Eating does not have to satisfy only the physical, it can do so much more for you – as long as you understand that you truly are worth it. Then you can select your 'treats' from amongst those foods that you know will benefit you rather than harm you, and you can derive your 'comfort' from those foods that will indeed provide genuine nourishment.

Finally...

I understand your need for continued support – through the first stages of defining your personal goals, developing and implementing your personal plans, and maintaining your new habits and sustaining your fabulous changes FOREVER! So I'll be there. I want you to succeed. I want to help you to combat type 2 diabetes for good! **'the 6 diet'** provides all the information you need to succeed.

However, if you find working from a book a lonely journey, and would like to receive face-to-face support and guidance along the way then why not apply to be accepted onto a RebalanceDiabetes programme? You will find that RebalanceDiabetes is there for you every inch of the way, providing all the advice, resources and encouragement you need to gain and maintain your ideal body. We'll be there to help you get the best of the 25% of your food nourishment, working with you to make the best choices for you. We'll be there as part of the other crucial 75% too – as your friend, advisor and partner on your new lifestyle journey. Visit **www.RebalanceDiabetes.com** for more details.

I wish you good health, from my heart!

Elaine

'the 6 diet' can help you achieve the

health and weight you truly desire and deserve

RebalanceDiabetes will support you every step of the way.

Visit **www.RebalanceDiabetes.com** today!